Treatment Strategy for Migraine

An effective treatment strategy for migraine

By

Lynne D M Noble

Copyright 2018 Lynne D M Noble
Updated April 2023

This book shall not, by way of trade or otherwise, be lent, re-sold, hired out, or otherwise circulated without the prior consent of the copyright holder or the publisher in any form of binding or cover than that in which it is published and without a similar condition including this condition being imposed on the subsequent purchaser.
 The use of its contents in another media is also subject to the same conditions.

Independently published

About the Author

Lynne Noble was born in 1953 in Huddersfield, West Yorkshire. From a very early age, Lynne showed an interest in nutrition and genetics avidly reading any books that she could get her hands on at the time.

Initially, Lynne studied orthopaedics but events led her to work with the elderly mentally infirm. Here, her interest in neurodegenerative disorders and pain syndromes developed.

Lynne undertook rigorous programmes of study, completing her Cert Ed., (FE) BSc (Hons) and Adv. Dip Education simultaneously before moving onto her M.Ed.

From there she took further demanding programmes in Human Nutrition, Pharmacology, Neuroscience, Genetics and Immunology. During this time, she was given many prestigious awards for her academic work. It was noted then that Lynne was not afraid of tackling difficult subjects.

She began her law degree but ill health prevented her from pursuing this. However, in this time, she moved from being a foster parent to adoptive parent.

She has been instrumental in setting up projects in the community for disadvantaged groups.

She is a member of the Guild of Health Writers.

Now retired, she lives in a picturesque village in West Yorkshire with her husband. She enjoys gardening, watching her husband bowling and researching.

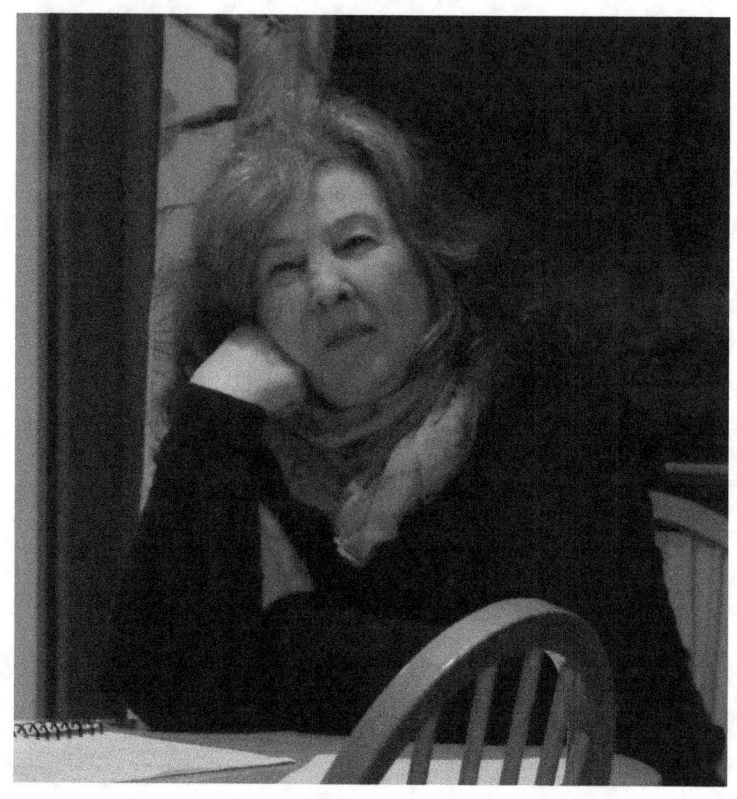

Author Lynne Noble at home

https://quintessentiallylynne.weebly.com/nutritional-medicine.html

Contents

A personal account – page 1

What is migraine   - page 9

What to do in the prodromal and

Initial (relaxation stage) of

migraine   -   page 17

Treatment strategy for a migraine attack page 28

The role of nitrates in migraine headache 47

Salt may cause/prevent migraine headaches page 51

The menstrual cycle and migraine page 53

MSG page 55

The fasting migraine headache, the breakthrough

 page 72

Migraine and vitamin B12 deficiency page 72

Riboflavin deficiency and migraine page 87

Abdominal migraine page 93

Curcumin page 124

Thiamine – the righter of all wrongs page 127

Dedication

To all migraineurs

A personal account

When I was a child, I distinctly recall my mother complaining of a 'sick headache' and taking herself off to bed to lie in a darkened room. I don't think that I'd ever had any type of headache at the point and didn't really understand what was going on. I suppose children can be a little unsympathetic but it was a little hard to have to tiptoe around for a few days until my mother had recovered.

I did not suffer from migraines until I had my first child. That was the beginning of relentless migraines which blighted my life. I began to dread having periods since the migraines would start two days before their onset and continue for four or five days. I began to dread sunlight since that would set it off. I began to dread any stressful event – and believe me, I had plenty of those – for that would set the migraines off. I could not eat chocolate otherwise my head would be pounding the following day.

Migraine makes you feel distinctly unwell. It impacts your whole life with pain which is pounding in your skull without respite. The nausea rises up and is overwhelming in its intensity. It did not matter if I starved myself or ate. The migraine continued until it was spent. Even when it started diminishing I was left feeling utterly wrung out but grateful that I would have a few days of 'normality' before it would start all over again.

Was I capable of parenting at those times? No, I wasn't even capable of looking after myself as I lay in a darkened room on pillows which, at those times, appeared hard and unyielding. I could not cope with noise or light or any demands made on me at all. I was hard on myself. I dragged myself into work. I had a responsible job and a couple of 'duvet days' wasn't an option for me. It's difficult to explain to people who don't have migraine exactly how debilitating the pain and nausea is. For me, it is the worst physical pain I have ever experienced.

My mother's migraines stopped when she entered the menopause. At last there was some hope for me. I spent most of my young adult working life wishing for that magical stage in my life when my migraines would simply cease to exist. The reality is that I had migraine post menopause but not with the intensity that I had in my youth. However, they still had the power to make me feel very ill indeed. The only good thing now was that once I retired, I was not responsible for client welfare or parenting children so I could take time out without the feelings of guilt that so often accompanied the migraines when I was younger.

I did visit the GP, initially, since ibuprofen and paracetamol did not deal effectively with the pain. The feelings of nausea – which often ended in vomiting – and just general 'yukiness' did not respond to it at all. I was young and active. I did not need this 'thing' in my life disrupting it every few days.

I was given Migraleve which was only partially effective. Following on from that I was prescribed Zolmitriptan. This took the pain – if not the nausea – away for a whole half hour. It had peculiar side effects. My back went into spasm every time that I took it. This meant that I not only had the headache and sickness; I also had back spasms, too.

Sometimes, I had auras. These were like multi-faceted diamonds in the form of an arc in my central line of vision. They always preceded the pain when I did have them. They only lasted for about 20 minutes. I didn't have them often when I was a young adult but I do now. They sometimes occur now and are often not followed by the pain of a migraine headache.

I was involved in quite a bit of research at the time my migraines peaked. The research was enjoyable: not stressful. It did not contribute to my migraines but I used this skill - and the motivation that unbearable pain can give you - to investigate the underlying processes governing the headache.

I identified that my migraine headaches occurred:

- After drinking cocoa and eating chocolate – the darker the chocolate the quicker and more intense the headache
- Prior to a monthly period
- In response to bright light
- Stress
- Staying in bed longer than I normally would even if it was only half an hour more
- Missing meals

At one point, I always had a migraine on a Saturday afternoon, shortly after I had finished teaching. (I taught privately). I thoroughly enjoyed teaching and did not find it stressful. My Saturday pupils, who were being tutored for entrance exams, were an absolute delight. This pattern of teaching and then finding I was incapacitated with migraine for the rest of the weekend was a puzzle.

In the end I figured it out when I realised that the sunlight was hitting the polished table and reflecting it back into my eyes. After that revelation, I covered the table with a cloth and never experienced a migraine again after I had finished teaching on a Saturday afternoon.

I always found sunlight difficult to cope with, too. I have to carry a large pair of sunglasses around with me in order to avoid a migraine.

Knowing the triggers for my particular migraines did not always help me avoid them. Taking the pill did not change the pattern. I had a responsible job and could not always take meals at set times. I could avoid chocolate but I never quite came to terms with the fact that a migraine would always occur after eating even a small piece. Every so often I would try a piece, if offered to me, and pay for it during the early hours of the morning.

Stress and three children went hand in hand. There were lots of stressors in my life and most of them were unavoidable.

I wasn't just interested in the triggers, though, I was also interested in the processes underpinning the headache. What was going on? What had eating chocolate got to do with being unable to bear bright light? Was there a connection that I wasn't aware of. I scoured research papers on migraines. They did not reveal a great deal. Most of the research I came across appeared to be as confused and uncertain about migraine as I was. It was groping in the dark and hoping that something of some use would be pulled out.

I still do not think that migraine is given the place it deserves in research given the amount of pain and loss of quality of life, which is considerable. For me, it was and still is, the worst pain that I have ever had to endure. A little phased by the lack of any really useful research on the causes of migraine, I concentrated on the other studies that I had at the time. I only returned to look at migraine again when my daughter and youngest son, also began experiencing them. It is difficult seeing those you love in pain and feeling utterly helpless in addressing their pain. My son was placed on prophylactic medication but this did not work, either.

I had at that point discovered magnesium. I cannot recall how I 'discovered' that it could be useful for migraines but I bought some. I took 400mg at the onset of a migraine. Strangely, the pain did not manifest itself although the feeling of being utterly ill and nauseous did continue. I did not mention this to my daughter but I did give her some magnesium to try. When I saw her later she reported that the pain had not developed but she had still felt nauseous. Now, I know that this is not much of a study but I had not told her how it had affected me yet her experience was exactly the same.

At that point I really had to start at the beginning and ask myself this question.

What is migraine, exactly?

What is migraine?

I thought I was having a stroke. I couldn't see, couldn't bear the light. It kept flashing and bits of my vision had disappeared entirely. The colour had disappeared from some of the objects which I could still see. It was surreal. My arm did not feel as though it belonged to me. The side of my face was numb. Within half an hour, the pain started, like no pain that I have ever experienced. It was deep and thudding penetrating my brain relentlessly. I truly wished the ground would open up and swallow me.

A migraineur

A migraine is totally different from a 'headache.' A migraine attack can start hours or days before the actual headache begins. This is called the prodromal stage and it is often characterised by food cravings, fatigue, euphoria and excessive yawning. I also had excessive anxiety without any external reason why this should be so. Prior to the headache an aura may also occur. This consists of flashing lights, visual

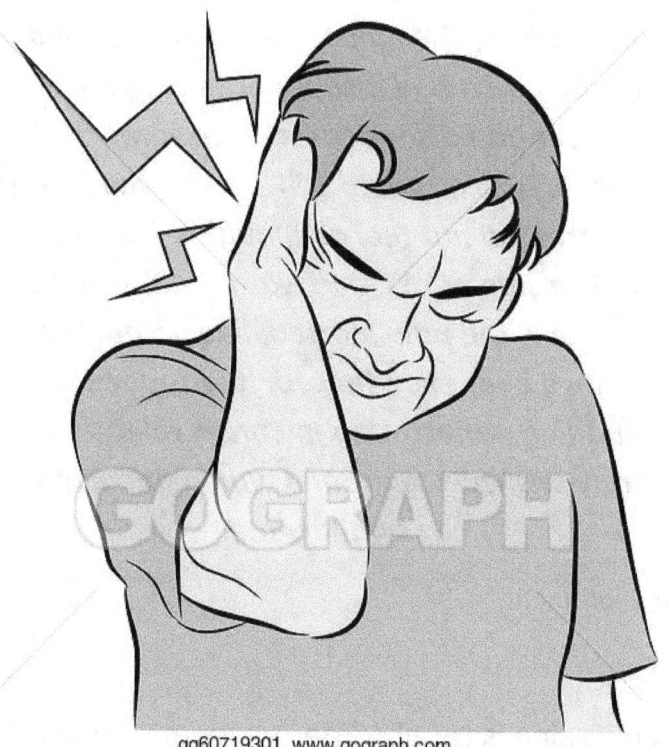

hallucinations or smells. The headache when it does occur is intense and throbbing. It may last for days. It may be accompanied by nausea and vomiting. Its severity is such that sufferers cannot work or think clearly.

The cause of migraines is believed to be due partially to the state of the blood vessels in the brain. The aura appears to be due to a phenomenon called 'spreading depression' in which there appears to be a loss of activity in groups of nerve cells in the brain. This loss of function spreads and is accompanied by a reduced blood flow through blood vessels in the brain.

This stage is followed by relaxation of the blood vessels. When the blood vessels relax, the nerve endings in the blood vessel walls become stretched and damage them as they are extremely fragile. As the nerve endings stretch they will cause pain.

However, this isn't the only cause of the pain. Once the nerve endings are stretched, they set off the release of several chemicals which are associated with tissue damage and inflammation. As the inflammatory action grows, the released chemicals cause the blood vessels to become leakier so that more substances gain access to the nerve endings and increase the pain even further. Mast cells are immune cells which are involved in the acute inflammatory stage of an immune system response. They release histamine and more pain producing peptides. It is not surprising that migraineurs often have allergies or that anti-histamines can address some migraine headaches.

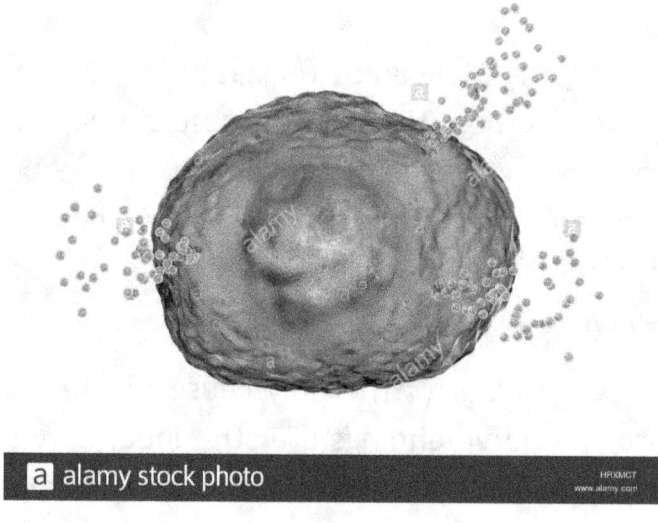

Mast cell releasing histamine.

When we look at the underlying process of migraine headache and of an 'ordinary' headache. This is what we see.

Normal headache	Migraine headache
Stress/tension induces muscle contraction which damage cells and activates cyclooxygenase and the production of prostaglandins.	Migraines occur as the nerve endings are stretched after being relaxed. Pain messages are sent to the brain, as a result. When the brain cells are stretched, inflammatory mediators such as histamine, 5HT, prostaglandins and peptides are released. This increases the sensitivity to pain.
NSAID's such as ibuprofen reduce the formation of prostaglandins	• Antihistamines treat histamine release • NSAID's reduce the production of

	prostaglandins • Ergots contract the blood vessels • Using beta blockers to stop calcium entry into blood vessels, which prevents contraction of the blood vessels as does magnesium.

Diagram showing a) normal blood vessel and b) leaky blood vessel during inflammation

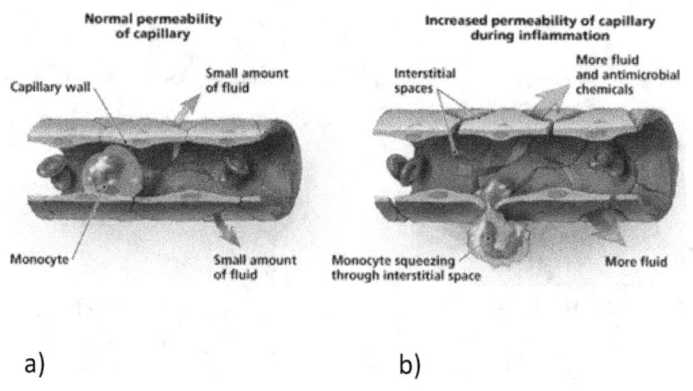

a)   b)

The pattern of events in migraine is:

Spreading depression – loss of activity in groups of nerve cells in the brain (aura stage)
Reduced blood flow through blood vessels
Relaxation of blood vessels and damage to nerve endings. This stimulation will cause pain.
Formation and release of a number of inflammatory mediators causing tissue damage and increased pain caused by the extra stretching
The leakiness is also increased so that more substances involve in leakiness can gain access to the blood vessel increasing the pain even further.

5HT is also known as serotonin. It can act on blood vessels and contract them. The 5HT-1 receptor seems to be particularly important in the development of migraine. There are a number of receptors for serotonin in the brain. One of the functions of serotonin is to contract involuntary muscle. This will reduce the blood flow to blood vessels thus preventing the relaxation of blood vessels which causes the nerves stretching. As such, intervention at this stage could abort a full blown migraine attack.

Sumatriptan was introduced by Glaxo in 1992 to deal with this stage of a migraine attack. This is why it was so important to take drugs like this which included

- Zolmitriptan
- Naratriptan

right at the beginning of a migraine attack before the dilatation stage has begun. This meant always having your medication with you so that the next stage of a migraine attack isn't reached. That is, the stage where inflammatory mediators flood leaky blood vessels.

As the medicines that activate 5HT-1 receptors, also cause contraction, they can also cause side effects which feel similar to angina such as pain and tightness in the chest.

Sumatriptan and similar drugs work on the blood vessels but they are also able to inhibit secretion of the inflammatory mediators to some extent. However, most people, who suffer with migraine, will state that these drugs do not always abort an attack even when given at the prodromal stage. I was such a person. Zolmitriptan only worked for half an hour before the pain came back. Taking another one at the prescribed time did not work either.

Once the inflammatory mediators have cascaded into action, then the migraine sufferer will begin to feel really ill. A multi-pronged attack is necessary at this stage because we are now past the stage when the ergot drugs (Sumatriptan and such like) are going to be effective.

As it is there is a much better way to prevent chronic low serotonin levels so that the relaxation of blood vessels, which causes the nerve stretching, does not occur.

What to do at the prodromal and initial (relaxation stage) of migraine

I had always wanted to be a teacher and a mother. I met Jed when I was twenty two and we married a year later. When I conceived I thought I was the luckiest person alive. Jasmine was perfect, dark-eyed and dark-haired like her father.

My migraines started about four months after Jasmine was born. I didn't know what they were at the time. I lay in a darkened room unable to attend to Jasmine's needs. I lay there listening to her crying. I rose half-heartedly, my head was pounding and I vomited on the carpet. I couldn't bend down to clean it up such was the pain. It was like a hammer going off in my head.

Eventually Jed came home and took over but, at that point, I was beyond caring.

When I had recovered I visited my GP and was informed that it was migraine. Of course, I had heard of it, but never could I have realised the impact that it has or has had since on my life.

I was given medication to take at the first sign of a headache. It worked only for a short time and, in the meantime I had to be a wife and a mother.

The migraine's normally started in the middle of the night. Jed got used to me getting up in the middle of the night to take my medication.

It's not just the pain, the period after the headache goes is just dreadful. I am drained, have no energy. My mother-in-law has to come and take Jasmine for me. Luckily, she lives close by. Heaven help those who do not have support like I have.

I eventually returned to my dream job, teaching. I found that I could not cope with the noise nor concentrate on teaching during my migrainous episodes. I know I was not the 'nice' Mrs S that the children once knew. I wasn't coping and eventually took extended leave. I am on a prophylaxis at the moment and I am awaiting an appointment to see a neurologist.

My life has changed considerably now. Jed and I had considered having three children at one time but I can barely cope with Jasmine although she is a dear, sweet child.

Yes, having migraine has changed my life considerably.

Sue, a migraineur

At the prodromal stage, eat some carbohydrate to increase the production of serotonin. This could be biscuits, brown rice or lentils.

Take your medication or supplements

If the migraine attack continues……….

In the early stages of inflammation histamine is released. I wish I had known this all those years ago before I studied immunology and found this out for myself. Histamine can make you feel truly awful. If I had known then that all I had to do was to take an antihistamine to address **one** part of the inflammation caused in migraine.

No one ever did. I have suffered years of pain because this one treatment wasn't suggested as an adjunctive medication. It could have helped considerably.

It is perhaps telling that I have a number of other conditions which occur due to histamine. These include

- Asthma
- Angieodema
- urticaria

as well as migraine. This should have raised warning bells as I have asthma, urticaria and angiodema. It didn't.

There is a condition known as histamine intolerance which is more widespread than is known or diagnosed. People have an intolerance to histamine. Its effects are systemic. When I look for the symptoms of histamine intolerance they include

- Headaches or migraines
- Nasal congestion or sinus issues
- Fatigue
- Hives/urticaria
- Digestive issues
- Irregular menstrual cycle
- Nausea
- vomiting[1]

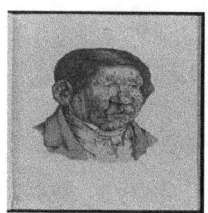

---

[1] https://www.healthline.com/health/histamine-intolerance

Histamine causes nasal congestion

In more severe cases of histamine intolerance these symptoms will appear:

- abdominal cramping
- tissue swelling (anywhere in the body)
- difficulty regulating body temperature
- dizziness

High histamine levels can be caused by:

- not enough of the enzyme diamine oxidase (DAO) which is responsible for breaking down histamine. There is DAO in olive oil, especially, if more DAO is needed.

- Medications that block DAO levels

- Gastrointestinal disorders such as leaky gut syndrome and inflammatory bowel disease.

- Foods which are naturally high in histamine which included any fermented foods

Prostaglandins are another substance of the immune system which cause pain. They respond very well to NSAID's such as ibuprofen. However, NSAID's are hard on the stomach. Fresh ginger also blocks the actions of prostaglandins

Some people take paracetamol which is not an NSAID. It acts in the central nervous system and is good at relieving pain. It can be taken alongside ibuprofen and an antihistamine. There are some people who cannot take NSAID's. For example, those with gastrointestinal problems and those on methotrexate.

Vitamin C, Magnesium and chronically low serotonin levels

Research suggests that magnesium is low in migraineurs and can lead to reduced blood flow to the brain and further, it is linked to low blood sugar levels. Both of these are implicated in migraine.

It is easy to see how missing a meal can start the cascade of events off for migraineurs. Most people are deficient in magnesium and missing a meal will just compound the problem.

Magnesium is useful because instead of taking the prescription beta blocker to stop calcium entry into the blood vessels which prevents contraction of the blood vessels, magnesium is a calcium channel blocker. As such it prevents the relaxation of blood vessels which cause nerves to stretch.

However, some people say that while magnesium does work sometimes it does not work all the time. We need to look into this further because clearly there is a reason for this

Vitamin C deficiency has not been implicated in the progression of a migraine but there are very real reasons why it should be considered more in the treatment of migraine as it appears to tie many factors that are involved in the progression of a migraine, together.

It is not well known that vitamin C is essential for allowing magnesium into the cells.

 Magnesium is an intracellular nutrient and simply cannot carry out its 300 functions in the body without being in the right place. Thus it cannot block calcium channels to prevent nerve stretching.

Vitamin C is essential for this so at the first sign of a headache then supplementing with 1000mg of vitamin C and 300mg of magnesium is wise. It really is not enough just to take magnesium if there is not enough vitamin C to transport it to the place where it can carry out its function.

As our diets vary on a day to day basis then it can be seen that, at times, a deficiency of either or both of these valuable nutrients can change the initiation or the manifestation of a migraine headache.

Vitamin C is a natural antihistamine and, as we have already seen, histamine is involved in the progression of migraine. Indeed, anyone with migraine and allergies should consider increasing their daily vitamin C intake either naturally or via supplements if this is not possible.

Vitamin C also regulates neurotransmitters like serotonin. It helps regulate the synthesis of serotonin as well as its release.

Vitamin C is also necessary for the conversion of dopamine to serotonin as well as helping to protect the neurons from oxidative stress.

Vitamin C is highly concentrated in the brain; indeed, higher concentrations are found here than anywhere else. Vitamin C is so important for brain function that the brain will attempt to keep sufficient levels even when the body is so depleted that over signs of scurvy exist.

Vitamin C is known to help alleviate depression and anxiety, characteristics of the mood changes found in the prodromal period of migraine.

All in all, it begs the question about whether migraine is just the manifestation of a vitamin C deficien

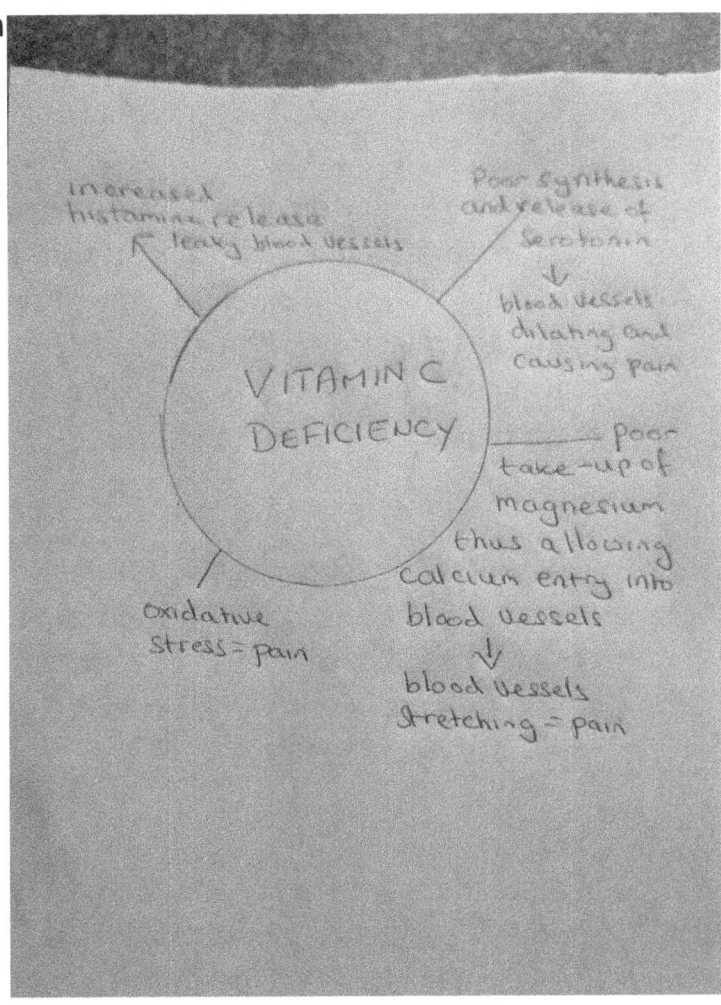

Low magnesium Iso appears to be linked with the menstrual related migraine but studies show that vitamin C is helpful in treating menstrual migraines through its ability to scavenge reactive oxygen species as well as attenuating brain inflammation.

Vitamin C attenuates excitoxicity via increasing the uptake of a neurotransmitter from the synaptic cleft and decreasing the activity of an NMDA receptor known to be involved in pain transmission.

Indeed, there are studies that suggest that vitamin C can be used prophylactically for menstrual migraines. One study found that 68.4% of participants saw at least a 50%

reduction in headaches after supplementing with vitamin C.

One wonders that, if this had been combined with magnesium whether the results would have been even higher.

We can now see that we can replace some of the medications that may be prescribed for migraine with more natural supplements so the original suggestions that doctors may put forward such as:

- 500mg of magnesium
- Antihistamine
- Paracetamol
- NSAID like ibuprofen.
- Prescription drug like Zolmitriptan

Could now be:

- 500mg of magnesium
- 1000mg of vitamin C (sodium ascorbate) which can be increased up to 5000mg over the day, if needed, as it will be used up very rapidly.
- Other supplements as appropriate which are mentioned later in this book.

This treatment strategy should deal with the pain very well. It is also likely to deal with the nausea and vomiting since this is most likely due to the histamine which has been released from the mast cells.

If, however, the nausea isn't dealt with then an anti-emetic can be added. However, increasing your intake of vitamin C should be a first consideration.

There are a number of anti-sickness medications which can be prescribed by your GP if the antihistamine doesn't work in alleviating the nausea.

The over the counter anti-emetics are Domperidone or Buccastem.

Domperidone is useful for vomiting caused by a bug or migraine. Its brand name is Motilium. It works by relaxing muscles at the entry and the exit of the stomach and increases stomach muscle contraction. This speeds the food through the stomach so there is nothing left in your stomach.

It also helps to prevent reflux as well as the messages which relay the feeling of nausea to the vomiting centre.

Buccastem, another over the counter medication, also prevents the messages, which relay the feeling of nausea to the vomiting centre, in migraine, as well as nausea due to stomach bugs and labyrinthitis.

Domperidone can be use up to three days running but Buccastem should be limited to no more than twice a week.

Domperidone is absorbed in the stomach and Buccastem is absorbed in the mouth. Buccastem, in this respect, has some advantages since it is efficiently absorbed

Unlike Domperidone, it is absorbed by the mouth, rather than the stomach.

'So if you are repeatedly being sick, it will still have the chance to be absorbed so it might be the better option if you are feeling very sick.

Antihistamines generally are very safe. The drowsy antihistamines will help you sleep off the migraine attack.

However, after stating all that we should consider the role of tryptophan which is an amino acid which, when depleted, enhances symptoms of motion sickness which includes: nausea and dizziness.

Now tryptophan is an amino acid that the body uses to produce serotonin. It is found in all animal proteins.

Tryptophan is a precursor to 5-HTP which is then converted to serotonin. It is of interest that I am able to abort a migraine headache just by taking supplements of tryptophan.

Vitamin D and the fatty acid, omega 3, found in fish, help activate the transcription of tryptophan hydroxylase 2 which synthesise serotonin in the brain.

Treatment strategy for a migraine attack

At the prodromal stage – take some carbohydrate like biscuits or a slice of toast. Take your supplements vitamin C and magnesium.

It is hoped that vitamin D levels are always kept within sufficient levels. It takes longer for these to build up although you could try 10,000 IU's at the first sign of an attack. However, it must be taken with magnesium which activates it and it must be taken with a little fat in order for it to be absorbed; it is, after all, a fat soluble vitamin.

Drink a cup of strong black caffeinated coffee. The caffeine in coffee constricts blood vessels so that they are less likely to go into the relaxation phase. There are a number of proprietary caffeine tablets on the market which you could carry around to form part of your rescue pack. However, some people have rebound headaches when taking caffeinated coffee or, indeed, any form of coffee. If this is you, miss the strong, black coffee or caffeine tablets out.

However, it is not only caffeine, in coffee, that helps prevent migraine headaches. Coffee also contains a substance call trigonelle. Trigonelle is a major active component of fenugreek and it has a number of beneficial properties other than helping prevent migraine.

Fenugreek is also called methi. The leaves and seeds are both used in Asian cookery. The freshly leaves are directly cooked like vegetables. Dried leaves and seeds are used in recipes like dhansak and daals. If you have chronic migraine, then it may help by introducing methi into meals if you do not already do so.

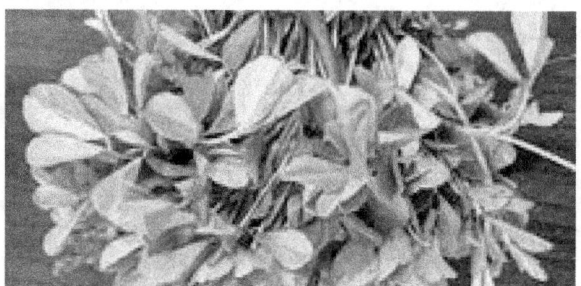

Fenugreek may help prevent migraine

Try and cool your body when a migraine begins. This will have the effect of constricting your blood vessels in order to avoid heat loss. You could try wrapping some ice cubes in a tea towel, or similar, and applying this to the back of your neck or to where your particular area of pain is.

If this doesn't work, or you think it probably won't, based on past experience, and the pain has started or you think it is about to start:

- **If you absolutely need to take antihistamines** – if your migraine comes on during the day and you have responsibilities which you cannot put aside then you need to take the newer antihistamines which are non-drowsy. However, if it is evening and you have a night's sleep in front of you, then take one of the older antihistamines like Benadryl, or Piriton, which will help you get a good night's sleep.

There might be a hangover effect, the following morning, with Benadryl but Piriton has a half-life of four hours in which case you will need to take another one or two after this period.

- **Magnesium 500mg**
- **500mg tryptophan twice daily if needed; it does induce sleep but is preferable to antihistamines.**
- **10,000 IU's vitamin D**
- **At least 1000mg vitamin C up to 5000mg**
- **Take anti-emetic if prescribed and needed (Domperidone or Buccastem can**

be bought over the counter). Vitamin B6 is also a good anti-emetic and is the preferred option. The recommended dose of pyrioxidine when used to prevent nausea and sickness is 400mg daily.

This rescue treatment is very effective. It goes without saying that you should carry this rescue pack around with you at all times and also keep one at the side of your bed – my migraines nearly always started in the early hours of the morning.

However, if you make sure that your diet contains adequate amounts of these valuable nutrients then this should keep even the beginnings of a migraine away.

While vitamin C and magnesium and pyridoxine (vitamin B6) works rapidly as they are water soluble vitamins, vitamin D will need time to build up to preventative levels.

Sometimes people are non-responders to vitamin D and it is necessary to add about 6 mg of boron to the diet which overcomes this problem

Preventing migraines

Sometimes when migraine sufferers have frequent and intractable migraine headaches, a prophylaxis may be prescribed. A prophylaxis is a treatment given, or action taken, to prevent disease.

Coenzyme Q10

Studies[2] have looked at the efficacy of coenzyme Q10 as a potential prophylaxis. Coenzyme Q10 is an antioxidant and occurs naturally in the body. It helps to generate energy in the mitochondria. Mitochondria[3] also protect cells from oxidative damage and viruses and bacteria that cause disease.

---

[2] https://www.ncbi.nlm.nih.gov/pubmed/11972582
[3] https://www.ncbi.nlm.nih.gov/pubmed/23065343

The study involved thirty-two patients – 26 women and 6 men) who had a history of episodic migraine with or without aura. They were given 150mg of CoQ10 daily. Only one patient failed to complete the study.

It was found that the average number of days with migraine during the baseline period was 7.34 but that this decreased to 2.95 after 3 months of therapy. This was a statistically significant response. Further, there were no side effects with coenzyme Q10. As such CoQ10 appears to have significant prophylactic properties.

As ageing progresses, coenzyme Q10 becomes depleted. However, a number of medications also interfere with the body's synthesis of CoQ10.

These include:

- Tricyclic antidepressants
- Haloperidol
- Statins
- Beta blockers
- Anti-diabetic sulfonylurea
- The anti-hypertensive clonidine

An alternative medication may need to be considered if an individual has regular episodic migraines.

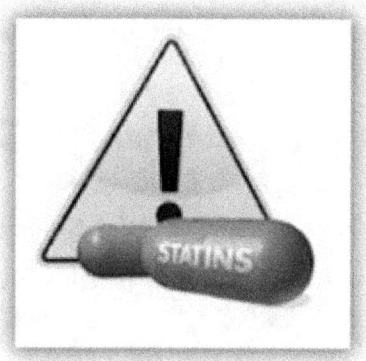

Statins may be a risk factor for migraines.

Good food sources of coenzyme Q10 (and tryptophan) are:

- Organ meats such as kidney, liver and heart
- Muscle meats such as beef, chicken and pork
- Fatty fish such as sardines, salmon, mackerel
- Nuts and seeds
- Legumes such as peanuts, lentils and soybeans
- Vegetables including spinach, broccoli and cauliflower
- fruit

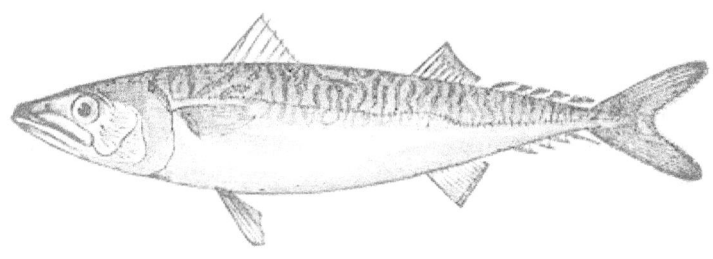

Mackerel is a good source of coenzymeQ10

Coenzyme Q10 can be obtained online or at most good health food stores, too.

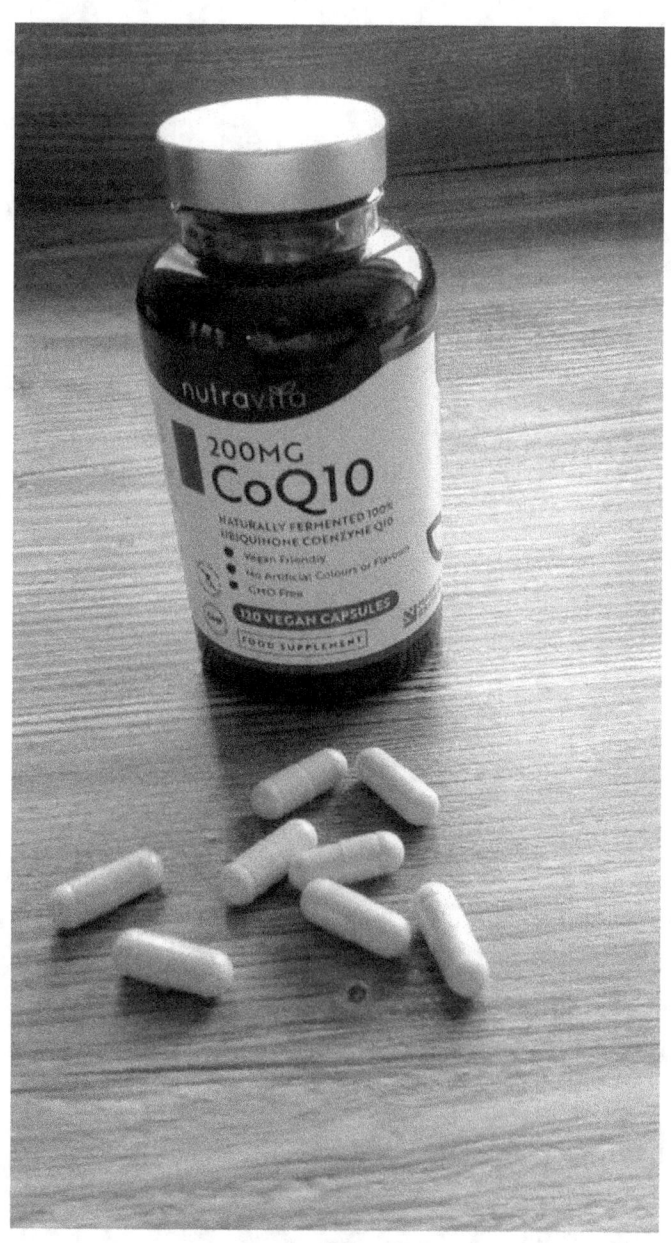

Butterbur

The University of Michigan conducted a study to look at whether the herb, butterbur, may reduce the inflammation that occurs in blood vessels during a migraine attack. The herb regulates neurotransmitters in the brain and appears to lessen the likelihood of migraine attacks.

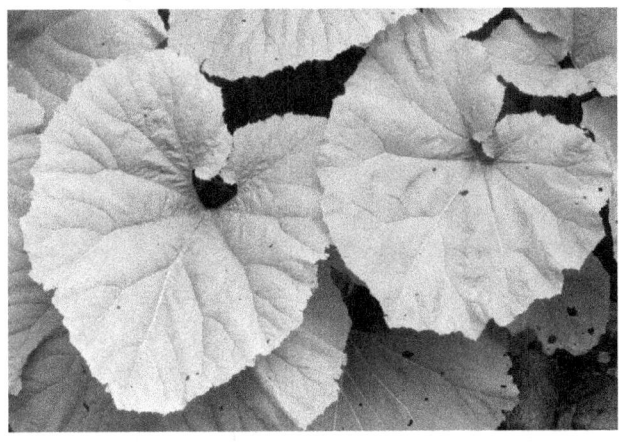

Butterbur has been found to lessen the likelihood of migraine attacks.

Melatonin appears to decrease the risk for migraines. A number of studies have found that when melatonin is given to migraine sufferers it helps to relieve pain and also headache recurrence.

What is melatonin? Melatonin is a hormone that is made in the pineal gland which is located in the brain. Melatonin regulates the sleep wake cycle and melatonin is influenced by the internal clock (circadian rhythm). The amount of light that you are exposed to also influences the amount of melatonin that is synthesised.

Natural daylight helps to produce and optimal amount of melatonin. This is because melatonin levels at night are dependent on a complete shutdown of melatonin during the day. The earlier in the day that this occurs the better. Any daylight is better than none but in order to maximise the amount of melatonin production at night, exposure to extremely bright sunlight during the day, is the desirable goal.

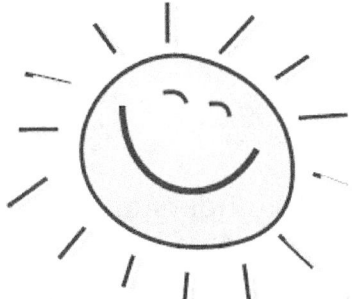

We have only to compare the light intensity – which is measured in luxes – of that produced in offices (approximately 400 lux) to that of the sun which is ten times greater during the day to realise that most of our working life is geared towards producing poor quality sleep. This does impact on our vulnerability to migraine attacks.

Most people report that they don't fully wake up in the morning until they have received some 'proper daylight' as opposed to the yellow light emitted by most light bulbs.

The very elderly housebound, who often complain of poor quality sleep, could very well be victims of the 'yellow light syndrome' since they are hardly ever outside to take advantage of the sun's effects on subsequent melatonin production.

However, it is important to understand that vitamin C is also necessary for the synthesis of melatonin. Remember, that I said that vitamin C helps the synthesis and release of serotonin, well vitamin C helps in the synthesis and regulation of many neurotransmitters.

Some groups of people who may suffer from sleep deprivation due to the lack of sunlight are

- the housebound, sick and elderly or even the very young

- office workers

- nurses, teachers, those working underground, shop workers, millworkers, among others

Alcohol has been found to interfere with melatonin production. While the initial effects of alcohol are to make you feel relaxed and drowsy its later effects are that it will wake you up a lot earlier than you wanted.

The relationship between melatonin and cortisol

Melatonin is, as we have seen, the hormone which regulates the sleep-wake cycle. Cortisol is a steroid hormone that is produced by the adrenal glands. These sit on the top of the kidneys. When cortisol is released into the bloodstream, it can act on many different parts of the body and help it to respond to stress or danger. Cortisol also helps increase the body's metabolism of glucose.

Cortisol is a necessary stress hormone that is designed to aid wakefulness in the morning as well as enable us to cope with danger. An increase in cortisol also triggers the release of amino acids from the muscles, fatty acids into the blood stream as well as glucose from the liver. This all helps us access an enormous amount of energy should we need it in an emergency.

Modern life does not allow us to burn up this amount of available energy with intense physical activity. The elevated levels of hormones continue to impact on the body and stimulate the release of even more stress hormones.

When I was teaching and the pupils were coming up to exam time, I used to tell them to run around a lot more than usual just to release all the tension from their bodies.

Many children who find some schoolwork difficult can become agitated and fidgety. They are not being naughty. It is a natural response to the elevated hormones caused by a stressful situation. Punishing a child for this will only worsen the situation.

When people have received worrying news, they can become very agitated and unable to sit still. This is due to the stress hormones circulating in the body.

Children suffer from migraine too and need to be taught how to relieve stress when it occurs.

Modern day live has been so inculcated into us that it is the norm that we have forgotten that many things which are part and parcel of our lives are stressors. These include

- driving
- constant noise
- constant light including the light which surrounds us at night
- too much going on – I find packed supermarkets particularly difficult.

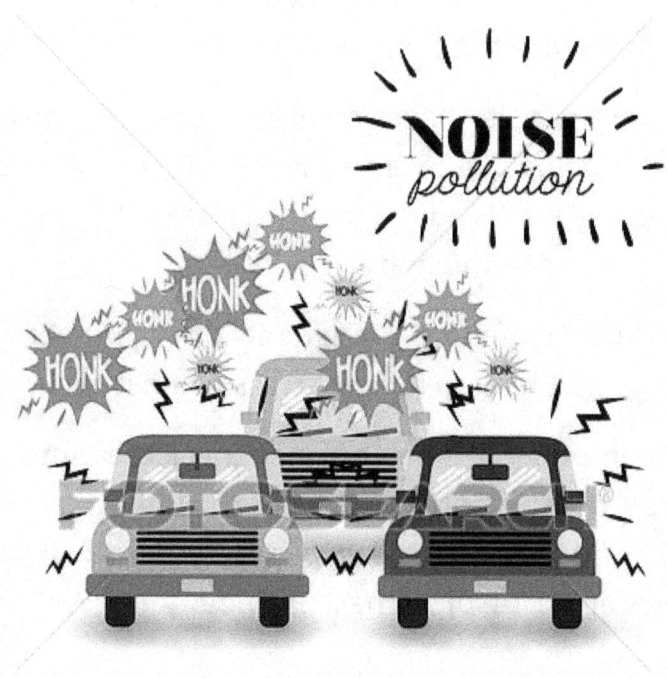

Cortisol has an antagonistic effect on melatonin. As cortisol rises, it correlates with a drop in melatonin and vice versa.

Studies have shown that physical stress decreases pineal melatonin levels at night whereas it increases melatonin production during the day. This is the opposite of what we want.

It is so important to identify the stressors which are impacting on good quality sleep so that adequate amounts of melatonin can be produced.

On a personal note, I have tried melatonin but this did not appear to be the underlying trigger for my own migraines.

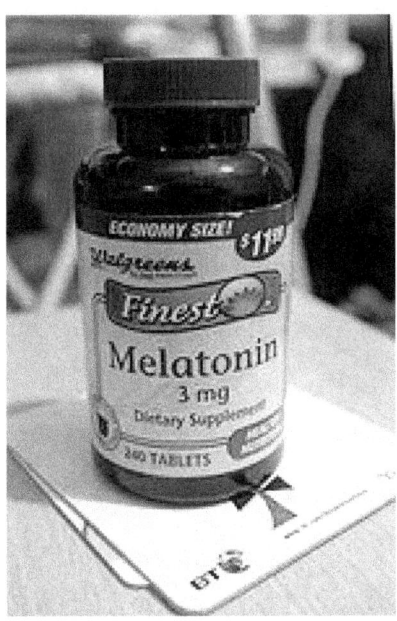

The role of nitrates in migraine headaches

Nitrates are chemicals that are found in the environment – in soil, water and air so they are ubiquitous. Nitrates may be added to food to stop the growth of bacteria. In addition, they also enhance the flavour of foods. Indeed, they are added to many foods to help preserve them. This is not good news for those who are predisposed to migraine headaches.

Nitrates are also used in some medications. Their ability to dilate arteries is useful in conditions such as angina where the pain of angina is due to narrowed arteries. Unfortunately, common side effects of nitrates include:

- Flushing
- Headache
- Dizziness
- Low blood pressure
- nausea

The American Gut Project research has found that migraineurs have higher levels of bacteria that are normally involved in processing nitrates. Eventually, nitrates turn into nitric oxide which are associated with headaches. As such, the above symptoms are likely to occur.

A theory known as the neurovascular theory, argues that vasodilation is not the cause of migraine headaches. They suggest that the pain is due to trigeminal nerve activation which stimulates fibres and elicits pain and inflammation in doing so.

If this is the case and it may be a cause for some people's migraines, then measures that are recommended for those who suffer MSG related migraine (see later in this book) may be a helpful treatment.

Nitrates are found in many foods including:

- chocolate – especially dark chocolate and cocoa
- bacon

- wine
- processed meats in general
- beets
- garlic
- leafy green vegetables
- citrus fruits
- nuts and seeds

Normally, medics encourage patients to include these foods in their diet as they help to lower blood pressure. However, for migraineurs this isn't practical given the impact on the migraineurs life. It may be that some of the above foods impact, more than others, on the potential to cause migraine. Most of the above, I have subconsciously avoided throughout my life, because the made me feel ill. However, I have never had a problem eating leafy green vegetables or beets.

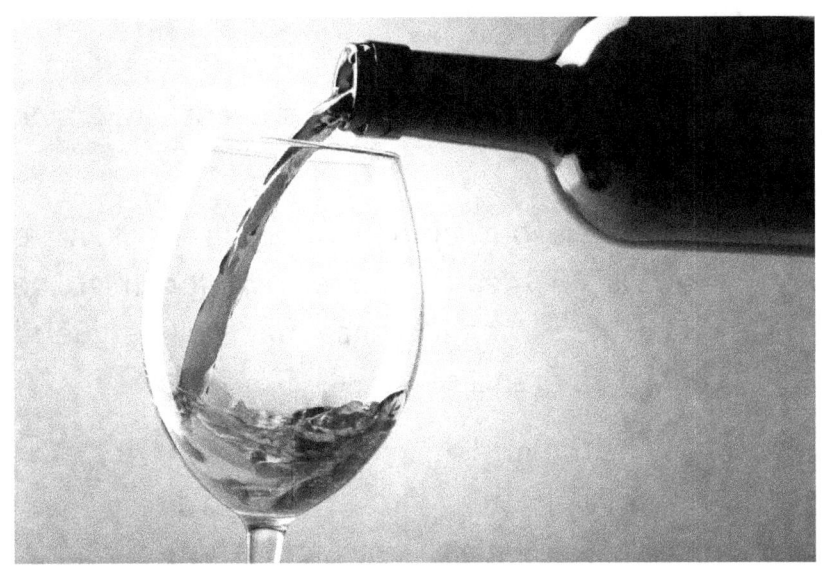

Red wine is well known for causing migraine

Salt may cause and prevent migraine headaches

The jury is out on whether salt is likely to increase or decrease the risk for migraine headaches. The difference may well be due to genetic differences.

A high sodium diet increases the risk for fluid retention and may prevent the twitchy blood vessels that initially constrict before dilatation occurs.

Research has shown that during a migraine, levels of sodium rise in cerebrospinal fluid.

Michael Harrington[4] at Huntington Medical Research Institute, California looked at the National Health and Nutritional Examination Survey that looked at the diets of thousands of people. Surprisingly, those with the diets that were highest in sodium were less likely to have migraine. This was surprising given that sodium

---

[4] https://www.newscientist.com/article/2101015-does-eating-more-salt-prevent-migraines-and-severe-headaches/

is known to activate neurons but it is believed that people with migraine handle sodium differently.

The findings by Harrington, have also been observed by Svetlana Blitsheyn of the University at Buffalo School of Medicine and Biomedical Sciences in New York.

Blitsheyn specialises in disorders of the autonomic nervous system and she observed that many of her patients suffered from migraine. If they consumed more salt, then their migraines often got better.

However, the diets the patients were on were typical high salt US diets. High salt diets are known to be associated to heart disease and strokes so caution is required before increasing salt in the diet to prevent migraines.

The Menstrual cycle and migraine headaches

Many migraineurs report that they have monthly headaches associated with their menstrual cycle. I was no different. Three days before my cycle started the familiar symptoms of migraine began and nothing I did to try and stop this, worked.

The migraines continued for a few days and then they would dissipate leaving me feeling like a wet lettuce for a number of days. I had three young, and lively, children to look after and this constant disruption in my life impacted me more than any other medical condition that I have had – especially as I had a short cycle which was normal for me.

Years have been taken out of my life because of this condition and, unless a medic has migraine themselves, they are unlikely to understand or appreciate the far reaching impact has on your life.

The hormone oestrogen drops before a period. If we produced oestrogen in the same amount around the month we would not suffer from menstrual cycle associated migraine.

One of oestrogen's wide ranging effects is to dilate blood vessels. Conversely, when oestrogen levels drop, blood vessels constrict initiating the first part of a migrainous cycle which may result in a migraine headache.

Magnesium is often recommended to be taken at the beginning of a migraine headache connected with the menstrual cycle. It has been found to be effective because it opposes the effect of reduced oestrogen. Magnesium dilates blood vessels and lowers blood pressure.

Not all migraine headaches appear to be directly related to twitchiness of blood vessels. Some amino acids cause neurons to become excitable and their potential to cause pain increases especially in susceptible people.

We shall now turn our attention to a major player in migraine, that of monosodium glutamate.

MSG

Monosodium Glutamate

Monosodium glutamate is the salt form of an amino acid. Glutamate is a very powerful neurotransmitter that is released in the brain by nerve cells. One of its functions is to relay messages between cells. It plays an important role in learning and memory.

For those susceptible to MSG —often found in Chinese cuisine - reactions can occur within minutes of it being ingested. Symptoms include:

- tightness and pressure around the chest and face
- excessive perspiration
- flushing
- restlessness
- a vague feeling of being unwell
- Swelling of the face, lips tongue

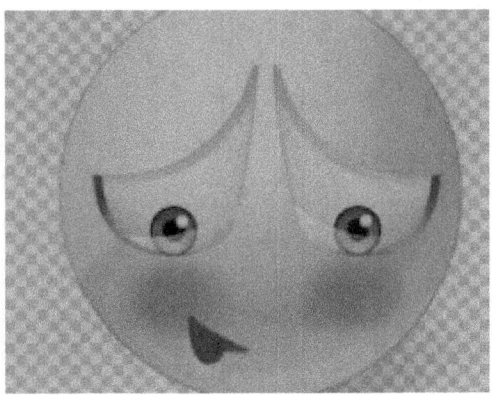

MSG can cause facial flushing

MSG is hidden in lots of foods and often not referred to as MSG. Look out for:

- soy sauce

- meat tenderiser
- hydrolysed protein – often found in stock cubes
- all natural protein
- sodium or calcium caseinate
- yeast extract
- gelatin

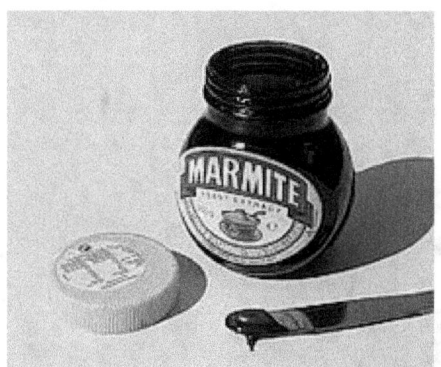

Yeast extract may induce migraines in susceptible people

The effects of MSG may be ameliorated by eating a diet high in complex carbohydrates such as potato, rice or pasta. Foods high in complex carbohydrates contain amino acids which are

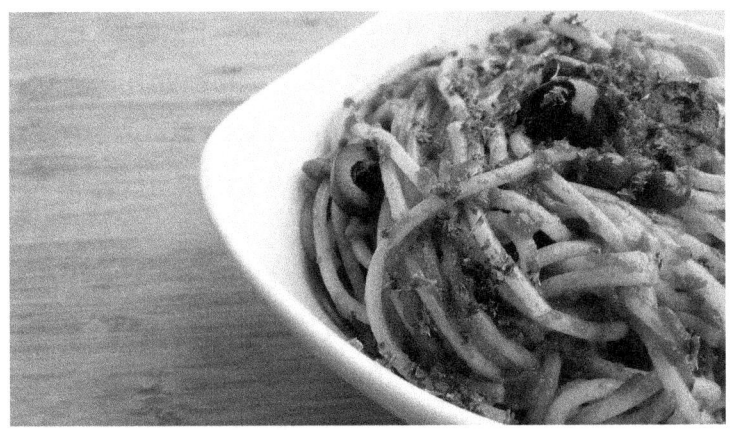
A small bowl of pasta may help prevent or ameliorate migraine if eaten early enough

inhibitory in nature and so calm down the brain cells which have been in an excited state.

Indeed, many patients who have migraines report that prior to the initial symptoms of migraine appearing they have a craving for carbohydrates. In a nutshell, they are subconsciously attempting to ameliorate the effects of MSG without understanding the reasons behind it.

Nevertheless, the benefits of complex carbohydrates in preventing migraine attacks extends beyond its treatment for MSG induced attacks. Carbohydrates naturally inhibit the firing of neurons that transmit pain. You can see why when people are anxious or stressed or in pain they turn to comfort eating. They are subconsciously addressing a need without realising how eating such foods is addressing the complex needs of the human body.

As soon as you feel a migraine coming on and before the nauseous feeling takes over it is always worth trying to eat some form of complex carbohydrate to see if it will help prevent or ameliorate the symptoms of migraine.

Some forms of carbohydrate that I personally have tried are:

- a portion of chips
- Biriyani or a milk pudding such as tapioca or semolina
- A couple of slices of wholemeal toast with preserve
- A dish of pasta

- A bowl of mashed potato (my favourite)
- A dish of lentil soup

All have been tried and tested and have helped me in controlling the duration and severity of my migraines.

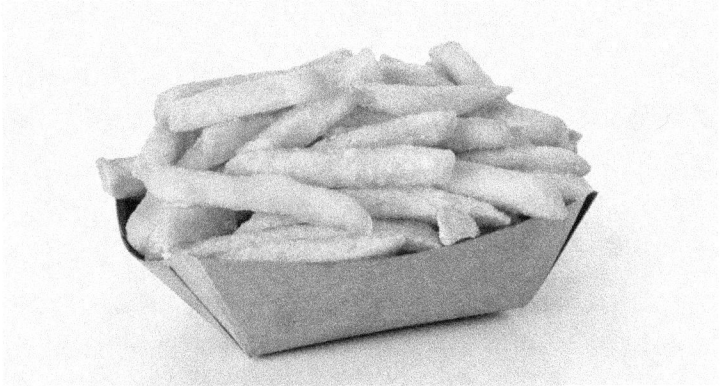

Chips are mainly carbohydrate and useful in controlling pain

However, the nutrient magnesium, that we have already looked at may also help with the pain caused by glutamate toxicity. It will help to understand why.

How does magnesium inhibit pain?

N-methyl -D-aspartate (NMDA) is a receptor for the neurotransmitter, glutamate. This means that a tiny part on brain cells is able to attach itself to a chemical called glutamate. Once glutamate has attached itself to the receptor it activates it. Glycine and serine, which are amino acids, may also activate the NMDA receptors.

When the NMDA receptors are activated they are associated with increased non-neuropathic pain, neuropathic pain and reduced functionality of opioid receptors. This means that the receptors that have an affinity for the pain killing opioids do not work as well. However, the level of activity on this this type of receptor varies.

Over activation of the NMDA receptor is relieved by magnesium as it causes a block on excessive influx of calcium ions that lead to excitotoxicity and increased pain levels.

However, it is important to preserve some NMDA receptor activity; we only want to remove **excessive** activity. In effect what is required is that the NMDA receptor is activated and then a channel blocker (also known as an uncompetitive receptor antagonist) blocks the flow of calcium ions that increase pain levels.

In medicine, the drugs ketamine, amantadine and memantine are prescribed. However, there are a number of natural NMDA receptor blockers and these include:

- parsley (contains agipenin)
- zinc (NMDA antagonist)
- garlic (s-aldyl cysteine)
- Dimethyl sulfoxide (DMSO) (an NMDA antagonist)

These substances are all found in local supermarkets or can be obtained in health food stores or online.

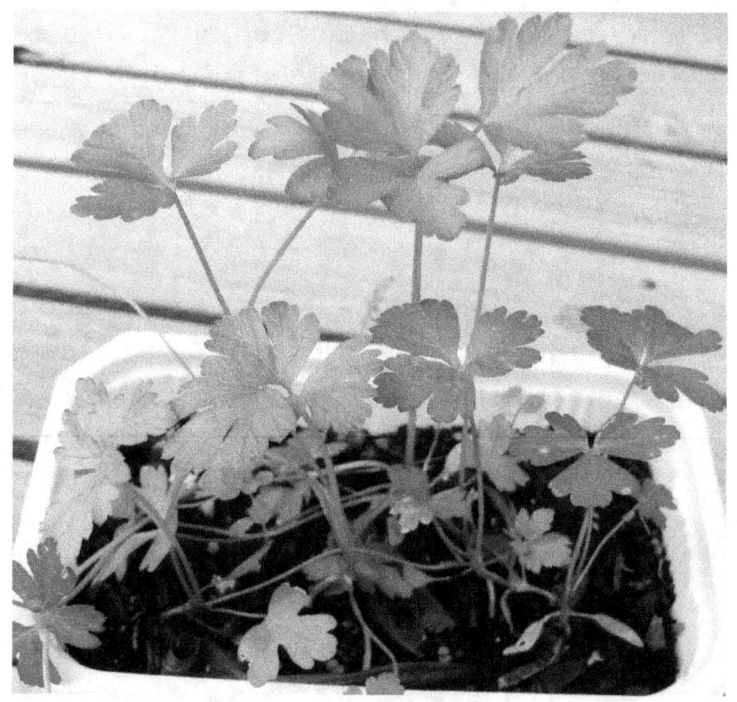
Parsley contains agipenin which may help to relieve the pain of migraine.

The Fasting Migraine Headache – the breakthrough

The fasting migraine is a commonly occurring experience for those who are on calorie reducing diets. Within two days of gently calorie reduction, the familiar signs of migraine appear. That generally ends the best of intentions when it comes slimming.

This is one aspect that never appears to be addressed at many support groups. It really needs to be.

It does not appear that 'trying to work through it' actually works. Six months after the birth of my second child, I embarked on a calorie controlled diet. I allowed myself 1500 calories so I did not cut calories drastically.

Within two days I started with a migraine. Fairly confidently, I started on my prescribed medication plus paracetamol and some ibuprofen. I did not respond.

I am fairly stubborn and so was determined to stick it out for a few more days but it did not dissipate. I continued for six weeks although how I managed it, I do not know. After that I gave up the gentle calorie reduced diet and the migraine slowly disappeared.

I never want a repeat of a status migraine again.

Over the years I have tried – and failed – to get a handle on this. Magnesium did help in attenuating the pain but not necessarily the feeling of utter lethargy and the ability to think or convey anything sensible.

My blood sugar levels did not appear to be involved. I ate a high protein diet with few carbohydrates in order that I did not have blood sugar spikes. It is these that help store excess calories as fat.

I also found it impossible to sleep when I was on a calorie reduced diet. I would lie there willing myself to sleep only to find that sleep evaded me. I would wake up feeling taut, miserable and looking gaunt.

Then one night the breakthrough came.

I had been researching tryptophan in some depth. It is an amino acid that is sometimes labelled as 'nature's prozac' and there is good reason why this is so. However, we first have to understand serotonin's connection with tryptophan.

Serotonin deficiency is implicated in:

- Anxiety
- Depression
- Insomnia
- Weight gain, among others

When the above manifest themselves and a serotonin deficiency is suspected then supplementation with serotonin directly cannot work. Serotonin does not cross the blood brain barrier.

Tryptophan is the sole precursor of serotonin but for synthesis of central serotonin to occur, tryptophan needs to cross the blood brain barrier. However, it is a large amino acid and when competing for the transporter system into the brain, the smaller amino acids hold the cards.

Further, most of the tryptophan that we do take in is generally bound to plasma albumin and therefore not available for transfer into the brain.

If tryptophan does make it into the brain, there are a number of enzymes which follow through a conversion process. Tryptophan is converted to 5-htp and through various other steps – all of which require various nutrients to be available - is eventually converted to serotonin.

The passage of tryptophan **requires carbohydrate** for it to be able to pass through the blood brain barrier. It is clear that during calorie reducing diets that not only is carbohydrate reduced but that many of the vitamins and minerals required for the conversion process of tryptophan to serotonin are unlikely to be available in the required amounts.

The anxious agitated state that may accompany migraine in the prodromal state is addressed by increasing tryptophan. This helps serotonin to balance the effects of two other neuro chemicals – norepinephrine and dopamine – which result in agitation and anxiety.

If, however, the depressive state results in apathy then tyrosine would help lift the mood as it is the precursor to dopamine and norepinephrine.

Many migraineurs have to be very disciplined with diet – missing a meal or a delay in one, can also bring on a headache - but there is a tendency to overeat with many migraineurs and the reason may be very simple.

Serotonin is associated with how we perceive hunger and fullness known as satiety. We know for example that excessive intake of carbohydrates helps increase serotonin levels so that tryptophan is able to act as an appetite suppressant.

A simpler method of reducing calories without risking a migraine is to increase vitamin C (and possibly magnesium) since vitamin C aids the synthesis and release of serotonin which is a natural appetite suppressant.

Further, vitamin C aids the oxidation of fat so that it can be used as energy.

As we have seen it is not that easy to get tryptophan to cross the blood brain barrier and, if we are trying to lose weight, we don't appreciate having to eat more carbohydrates in order to increase serotonin levels. However, you could try increasing foods containing vitamin C and tryptophan.

Foods containing tryptophan include:

- Turkey
- Tinned tuna
- Cottage cheese
- Oats
- Nuts and seeds
- Cheese

- Milk (milk being one of the largest sources of tryptophan)

However, for some people this will still not supply enough tryptophan to prevent a migraine, sleep disorders or the need to keep munching on carbohydrates until the migraine has dissipated.

Supplementation can then be considered.

Tryptophan can be obtained at health food stores and online. It comes in tablets or powder form. It has a slight flavour to it but it is not unpleasant.

The RDA for tryptophan is around 1gm but the small measuring scoops that come with the powder form hold 3g. For those prone to migraine this may be the best dose when they feel a migraine coming on, can't sleep or are embarking on a weight reducing diet.

People with a susceptibility to migraine appear to have a vulnerability in the serotonergic system. This may be due to a genetic susceptibility since migraine does appear to run in families but there may be other concomitant reasons that are, as yet, unknown.

Given the number of stages required for conversion of tryptophan to serotonin as well as a small amount of carbohydrate to aid tryptophan's transport across the blood brain barrier, a good varied diet taking in all the food groups is vital.

My bag of tryptophan cost £7.99 and will last me for approximately 8 months. That is such a small price to pay for the benefits it gives.

Migraine and vitamin B12 deficiency

Increasingly, the role of vitamin B12 in the prevention and treatment of migraine is becoming known.

Vitamin B12 is also known as cobalamin, cyanocobalamin or methylcobalamin and is responsible for a condition known as pernicious anaemia where the body cannot properly absorb vitamin B12 due to a lack of intrinsic factor protein. However, most cases of vitamin B deficiency are due to weak stomach acid – something that occurs in the elderly. There has to be enough stomach acid to separate the vitamin from its protein source in order for it to be absorbed.

A lack of vitamin B1 (which is required to release acid from gastric cell) is also a reason for poor stomach acid. Vitamin B1 is quite a vulnerable vitamin and is easily degraded by:

Drinking coffee or tea

A high carbohydrate diet

Alcohol

Some medications like Metformin or the proton pump inhibitors, like Omeprazole, also inhibit vitamin B1 from being absorbed. Omeprazole by virtue of reducing stomach acidity will also prevent the absorption of vitamin B12.

Poor diet can occur as a result of many factors. Plant based diets do not contain vitamin B12 which has to be supplemented from animal protein sources.

Birth control pills can also cause deficiencies in many of the essential vitamins and minerals. These include:

Vitamin B6, folic acid, vitamin C, magnesium, zinc

As well as vitamin B12.

The elderly are unable to absorb nutrients from food as well as they could when younger. Appetite is likely to reduce so that fewer nutrients are ingested. They need dense nutrition but often are unable to eat sources of these, like red meat, due to poor dental hygiene which may cause soreness. Many of the B complex when deficient will also result in sore mouths and tongue.

Therefore, any individual who has a propensity to migraine may find that it occurs throughout life but that the reasons for its manifestation may change over that period.

A negative correlation has been found between the serum levels of vitamin B12 and the incidence of migraine.

Vitamin B12 is needed to prevent hyperhomocysteinaemia which is known to cause cell damage in the endothelium when free oxygen radicals are increased. It is thought that it is this process that causes the onset of migraine.

Homocysteine is a protein which is required to fulfil a fleeting role in the body. It quickly gets broken down if there is enough vitamin B6, B12 and folate in the diet.

In the absence of the above, then homocysteine can cause considerable damage as it is highly inflammatory and causes a build-up of plaque in blood vessels.

It is recommended that migraineurs have regular check-ups in relation to their vitamin B12 status as well as attention to the other B complex which work in harmony with vitamin B12.

The deficiency symptoms of vitamin B12 which may well accompany migraine are

Smooth sore tongue

Nerve degeneration causing tremors, psychosis, mental deterioration

Menstrual disorder

Hand pigmentation (people of colour only)

Typical symptoms of anaemia

The best food sources are:

Pig's liver

Pig's kidney

Fatty fish

Pork

Beef

Lamb

White fish

Eggs

Cheese

Yeast flakes are generally fortified with vitamin B12 for those on a plant based diet. Yeast flakes are an excellent source of the B vitamins and do not have an unpleasant flavour when sprinkled over food or stirred into cooked soups or stews on being served. However, there is not always great amounts of vitamin b12 unless they are fortified so read the packaging to ascertain whether reasonable amounts of vitamin B12 are contained within.

The recommended intake is 3mcg daily but much higher doses of vitamin B12 can be taken without any problems whatsoever. It is always worth trying a month of 1000mcg daily to ascertain any impact on your migraine

Vitamin B2 deficiency and migraine

Many of the B complex vitamins are involved in reducing the risk of migraine but vitamin B2-riboflavin – is fast becoming known as a treatment in itself.

Riboflavin functions as a coenzyme flavin mononucleotide (FMN) and Flavin dinucleotide (FDN) which are needed to convert protein, fats and carbohydrates int0 energy. It is also used by the body to repair and maintain bodily tissues as well as mucous membranes.

In conjunction with vitamin B6, it also helps in the conversion of tryptophan to nicotinic acid.

As we have already learned, high amounts of homocysteine in the blood may contribute to migraine. It has been found that taking supplemental riboflavin for 12 weeks, decreases levels of homocysteine by up to 40%.

High homocysteine levels occur in people with who take medications for seizures. When riboflavin is taken with folic acid and pyrioxidine it can lower homocysteine levels by nearly 30%.

Riboflavin appears to work by enabling mitochondrial energy production. The mitochondria are tiny organelles within cells that are responsible for the production of energy. Imaging techniques suggest that disturbances in the mitochondrial metabolism in the brain occur in migraine patients. Further, migraine does share some symptoms with some mitochondrial disease.

The vasodilation and vascular dysfunction are partially addressed by riboflavin where 400mg has been taken for three months after which a break should be taken.

Deficiency symptoms which may accompany those prone to migraines include:

Insomnia

Difficulty in learning new material

Bloodshot eyes

Dizziness

Trembling

Hair loss

Tired eyes which are sensitive to light

Cracks and sores at the corner of the mouth

Inflamed tongue and lips

The stability in food is poor. It is easily destroyed by light. As such, riboflavin is normally kept in tinted glass bottles.

A deficiency of riboflavin is caused by alcohol, tobacco and the contraceptive pill.

The best food sources are yeast extract and dried brewer's yeast, liver, wheat germ, cheese, eggs, meat, yogurt and milk. However, sources of yeast are also sources of nitrates and may not suit everyone.

When I was a child, milk was delivered in bottles to the doorstep and placed on the doorstep with a cover over it; this so that if it wasn't taken in quickly would prevent the destruction of riboflavin which takes place rapidly.

Nevertheless, riboflavin deficiency was rife then. It was not unusual for me to observe the cracked corners of the mouths and rashes down the side of the nose which indicated a riboflavin deficiency. It appears more in the elderly now, most likely due to depleted appetite, poor absorption and disinterest in cooking.

Many people's migraine tends to go away after the menopause although some people do say the headaches don't appear but they still get auras.

It is important to realise that being prone to migraines at whatever time of life when they occurred is a risk factor for stroke so it is important to pay attention to the nutrients which are vital in eliminating the risk.

While I have evidenced that certain B vitamins can address the underlying issues in some migraines, it must be remembered that the B vitamins work synergistically and if you take one in therapeutic dosages then it is judicious to take a B complex in order to support the therapeutic vitamin.

For example, pyridoxine may be useful for nausea in migraine (and morning sickness) but it is not activated without the presence of riboflavin.

Following on from this pyridoxine is needed for the synthesis of dopamine which is then converted to serotonin. The importance of a varied and nutritious diet cannot be underestimated in tackling migraine. It is a horrible condition which can destroy lives and rarely responds in any great depth to prescription medicines which have some unwanted side effects.

To take the innocuous paracetamol we understand that the end product of metabolism is phenacetin which was banned as it was a risk factor for dementia.

Ibuprofen is well known for causing ulceration of the gastro intestinal tract but vitamin C helps heal any ulceration as well as thickening the mucus lining which forms a better protective barrier.

.

Abdominal Migraine

Abdominal migraine is often seen in children and less so in adults. It is clear that migraines cause gastrointestinal symptoms which may include pain, constipation, diarrhoea and nausea.

Maybe these are symptoms of food tolerance which is also associated with migraine or maybe some are associated with low serotonin levels.

Both migraine and constipation are associated with low serotonin levels. Vitamin C, of itself, outside the condition of migraine inducing constipation, can easily alleviate constipation. Most people are aware of vitamin C and bowel tolerance where increasing amounts of vitamin C are given every 1-2 hours until the bowel empties its contents with a watery whoosh.

After reading this book you should now be aware that vitamin C increases the synthesis and release of serotonin which helps move bowels. Most serotonin is stored in the bowel and not in the brain as is generally thought. In fact 90% of serotonin is made in the gut.

Your gut is more than capable of increasing serotonin release when required provided it has the necessary nutrients to do so. While we have recommended dietary intakes, they can only be a guide and there are many who can manage on far less than the recommended dietary allowance and just as many more who need much more than the recommended dietary intake.

If an abdominal migraine occurs with constipation, then taking approximately 200-

300mg of magnesium plus 3000mg of vitamin C initially increasing by 1000mg every hour or so may well shorten the episode.

When the vitamin C is working you will hear a rumbling in your stomach which will evidence that it is working. This rumbling tends to lessen as we age which probably reflects the lack of attention to the diet or the need to adapt it to the different nutritional needs of older age.

Some people experience a feeling of 'heaviness' in the lower abdominal area and to a lesser extent the upper abdominal area when they are predisposed to migraine but two or three days of high dose vitamin C (around 3000mg) can eliminate this. The feeling of heaviness is a good indicator that vitamin C levels are becoming insufficient for the job it needs to do.

Constipation as well as migraine is associated with psychological disorders such as anxiety and depression. Vitamin C deficiency is associated with both these manifestations of a mood disorder as well as fibromyalgia which is also thought to be due to low serotonin levels.

People with migraine or abdominal migraine tend to have greater bone density than those whose serotonin levels are well within levels to prevent migraine. This is because serotonin does affect bone density with higher levels a risk factor for osteoporosis. Bear in mind though that this is only a risk factor and not cause and effect.

Low serotonin levels are associated with many mood problems which can indirectly affect the gut. These include:

Insomnia

Suicidal behaviour

Post-traumatic stress disorder

Obsessive compulsive disorder.

Phobias

Panic disorders

The cause of low serotonin may not only be due to low vitamin C, although it generally is this or low tryptophan in diet, there is also the problem that some unfortunate people do not have as many receptors for serotonin as the majority of the population do.

Receptors are tiny shapes on cells that are specific for a certain substance. Without adequate receptors there are not enough 'hands' to grab onto the amount of serotonin needed.

Receptors do appear and disappear – a bit like a periscope – depending on prevailing conditions and the need for serotonin at the time but it still depends on environmental factors like essential nutritional availability and a relatively stress free life.

One of our most humble and popular vegetables, the potato, has fallen out of favour, yet is known as nature's Prozac such is its ability to contribute to serotonin levels. Potatoes contain high levels of vitamin B6, carbohydrate and potassium all of which contribute to proper levels of serotonin.

Potatoes, when cooked, become a form of resistant starch so that they do not contribute to high blood sugar levels which are a concern for some.

Indeed a bowl of mashed potato with butter and milk added may be the perfect natural remedy for any form of migraine provided extra vitamin c is taken.

Potatoes do contain vitamin c but how much is left once the potatoes have been cooked is debatable. Still it is time to put them back on the table and see them for the medicine they are.

Where serotonin can be increased then getting more tryptophan, sunlight, vitamin C and exercise as well as carbohydrate will certainly reduce the genetic risk towards this condition.

Note that high carbohydrate diets have a greater need for thiamine (vitamin B1) where thiamine converts them to energy. Thiamine is also required for the release of acid from the parietal cells in the stomach. This is important because poor acidity prevents the sphincter muscles from opening and closing to allow the contents of digestion onto the next stage or by preventing backflow into the oesophagus. It is quite possible that sodium ascorbate (vitamin C) raises acidity and allows a better flow of digested material.

In this respect it has a different function from that of synthesising and releasing serotonin. The human body is truly wonderful in its workings if looked after properly.

While outright constipation may not manifest itself, it would be unusual not to find some degree of gastroparesis where gastroparesis is a slowing of the digestive movement leading to bloating and other discomfort.

There are a number of common symptoms between migraine and slowed gut transit and these include:

- More likely to be found in women
- There is a link with Parkinson's disease
- There is a link with SLE
- There is a link with fibromyalgia
- There is a link with endometriosis as well as the mood disorders previously described.

While many medics can be quick to point out that these conditions are psychological in origin they do not always appear to realise that psychological conditions are embedded in nutritional deficiencies which, once treated, can disappear rapidly. Some of the treatments for migraine include anti-depressants, some of which will have long term disabling effects and do not appear to get to the root of the problem.

Metoclopropamide may be used to tackle both the headache and the gastroparesis. It is a medication which does speed up gastric emptying and is said to relieve pain. I have used metoclopramide decades ago and after 3 months decided I would not ever again. It gave me a peculiarly stiff posture and intense anxiety. It did not necessarily help the nausea or vomiting nor the banging headache which was constant so that the pillows felt hard and unyielding.

I decided that I did not want the migraine and the effect of the metoclopramide to go along with it. It may work for some people but I have not found anyone yet who believes it has. There is a particular sense that medics are struggling with treating migraine and are throwing anything at it in some desperation towards those patients who repeatedly set foot in the surgery hoping beyond hope that someone can do something.

I wish I had learned years ago what I know now. Then I would not have been unavailable to those who needed me when I was having an attack. I regretted passing it onto two of my children and watching them suffer – not that I did it on purpose but the guilt was still there all the same. No one wants to see their children suffer especially when you have experience of how deep that pain and suffering can be.

However, it did spur me on to look into the causes and effective natural treatment for migraine and abdominal migraine and it works. I know it works because so many people have come back to me to tell me so.

That is the silver lining in the clouds.

Final Thoughts

This book was written with the intention of empowering people to take control over their own pain. I am a migraineur and have spent a lifetime finding a treatment, which works, for a very debilitating condition.

I am sure that my children will long remember the days that I was confined to my bed or sitting in a chair feeling utterly miserable and hopeless unable to eat or cope with noise or any form of light.

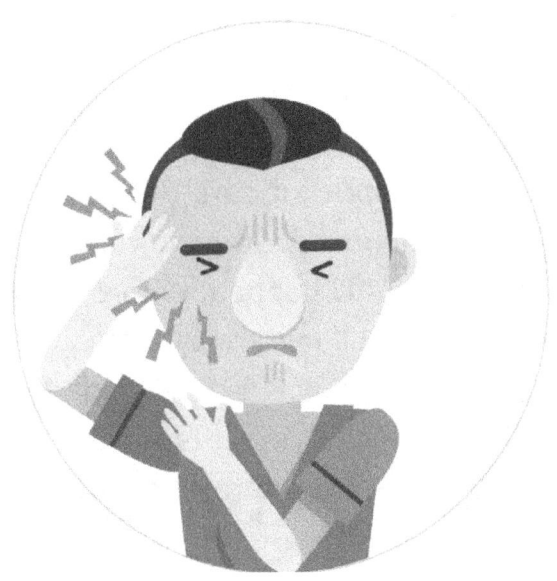

My pillow used to feel as though it was stuffed with bricks and, try as I might, I could never get comfortable. I would toss and turn all night with every movement a reminder of unbearable pain. A cold compress applied to the back of my neck might alleviate the pain for a short while but it did not relieve the nauseous feeling. If any medical condition can remind you of your fragility as a human being, migraine does.

In a way it regulates your whole life. If I stayed in bed for one extra hour at the weekend, then I would pay for it. One hour would equate to seven days of the process of having a migraine.

If I ate a couple of squares of dark chocolate or ate anything with monosodium glutamate in it then the same would happen. Even if I excluded everything I still had my monthly cycle to contend with. There was no escaping this familial condition which I inherited from my mother and which my daughter, unfortunately, inherited from me.

I learned as I went along. Zolmitriptan did not really work for me. It may have given me up to half an hours' relief but then the pain would come back.

In addition, the side effects of the medication just added insult to injury. My legs felt very stiff as though they did not belong to me. I did not need this when I was suffering already. I still had a household to run.

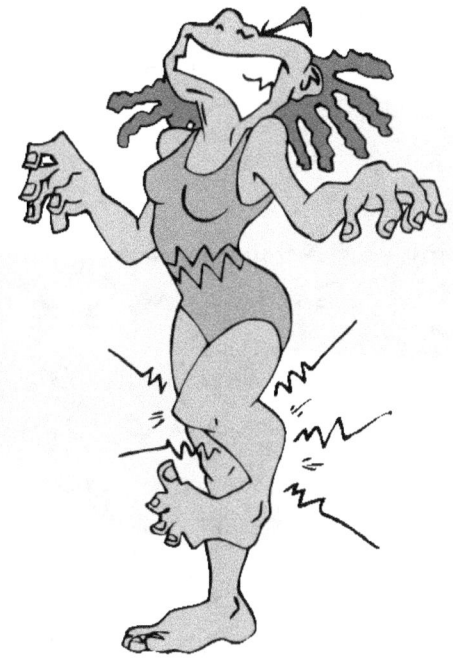

5

Zolmitriptan gave me stiff legs

I almost always turned down dinner invitations. One thing that I have learned is that migraine is not understood at all by those who are fortunate not to have it.

---
[5] https://www.clipart.email/clipart/sore-leg-clipart-72654.html

Given the regularity of my monthly cycle I could state without doubt if I would or would not be available to have lunch with someone well in advance of the invitation. Somehow, it does not seem right to say that you cannot make lunch in a fortnight because you will be experiencing a migraine then. It sounded like an excuse. I could understand another's disbelief on hearing this but it did not make it easier. I wanted understanding for myself.

I used to wonder how a condition that afflicts so many, is not taken more seriously. A population based study[6] found that work effectiveness was reduced by 41% for migraine headaches and by 28% for migrainous headaches.

I read this with some disbelief – only a reduction of work effectiveness of 41%? I was barely able to look after myself never mind contemplate the completion of any work related load.

---

[6] https://www.ncbi.nlm.nih.gov/pubmed/9633720

I did avoid certain foods because I learned that they made me feel ill. For years I had used an instant gravy when I was in a rush and did not have my own home made stock to hand. In time, I came to recognise that when I used this all in one instant gravy I became flushed and irritable and unwell. It did not surprise me to find out, many years later, that it contained a form of MSG. Who would have thought that of hydrolysed protein?

Then there was that vegetarian kick I went on. I bought quite a number of packets of textured vegetable protein and enthusiastically set about showing the children how to make interesting meals from a non-meat source.

I have to state that they did indeed taste good and I enjoyed the challenge of creating new dishes but I felt really ill during that time. Once I had removed the textured vegetable protein from my diet, I felt much better

Hindsight is a wonderful thing, isn't it?

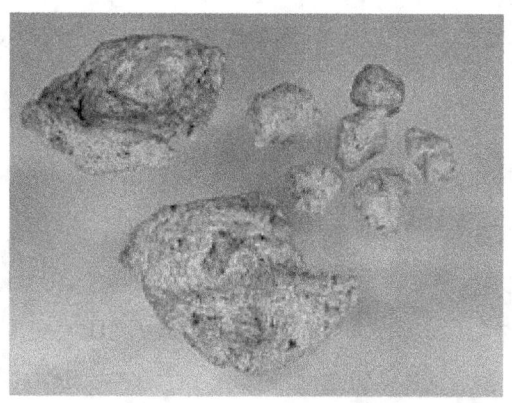

Textured vegetable protein can be a risk factor for migraine.

Many ready-made meals have TVP and hydrolysed protein added to them. It bulks the meat base out at a much cheaper cost but most people who sell them in cafes do not appear to have much idea of what goes to make up their meals.

It was much simpler finding out that chocolate could induce migraines within a couple of hours of eating it but perhaps it was not so simple to understand that this would be for *life*. Every so often when I was feeling well, I would try a square or two only to be reminded hours later that chocolate was definitely a 'no-no' if I wanted to avoid having migraine. In a similar vein I have had to pass on cocoa and drinking chocolate – both of which will induce a migraine within hours of consuming it. There are times, on a cold winter's day, when I am a little envious of those with a steaming cup of hot chocolate complete with miniature white and pink marshmallows. However, having migraine is a good teacher. I have quickly learnt aversions to food and beverage that will bring a headache on.

Likewise, my very first glass of red wine made me severely ill with a prolonged throbbing headache. I have never drunk any form of alcohol since. I cannot say that I miss it. Nevertheless, in some ways, it can be a little isolating at celebratory dos when I am the only attendee toasting with a glass of tonic water.

These measures did help a great deal but did not remove migraines entirely from my life. I had to avoid the reflection of sunlight off the water or the sun's rays streaming through the window. Even when I put blinds up a small chink of light would set them off. For a long time, I carried a pair of sunglasses with me all the time. Sometimes, when I was wearing them in winter, people would look at me strangely and some would comment at why I was wearing sunglasses in winter.

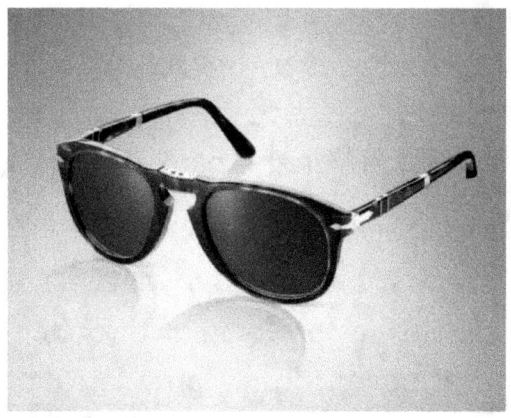

Sunglasses are a must for migraineurs

Eventually, these actions become habit so that you hardly notice the changes that you make even if they look odd to other people. If it was sunny I would walk with my head down even when wearing sunglasses. When we painted the house we always used matt instead of gloss paint. Colours were muted even though it may not have been my ideal colour scheme. All of these measures did help. However, it was at that point that I found that the smell of paint also induced a migraine.

My penultimate breakthrough - apart from avoiding known food and drink triggers – was discovering magnesium could reduce the pain if not the nauseous feeling. To some extent it liberated me, gave me hope but I was always looking further for the final cure. After that I realised that magnesium could not be effective without sufficient vitamin C and that really, for me was the breakthrough.

Prior to that I entered the menopause. Unlike my mother my migraines did not stop then but the hot flushes found me at my GP for relief. I was prescribed HRT – that, and pregnancy, had given me total relief. What a joy was that. Why did I have to reach more than half of my allotted life span to be afforded relief? It only lasted five years. Scares regarding HRT and increased cancer risk saw my prescription withdrawn.

However, my migraines were fewer and less troublesome. I did continue to get an attenuated form of one sided headaches but not the throbbing, banging sort that made even walking to the bathroom unbearable. I was still irritable and in pain but it was manageable.

Strangely, I could only ever recall having one aura with migraine prior to the menopause. Later I seemed to have an aura with migraine every time but this only happened once every six months now. Sometimes, the headache developed and sometime it didn't but at least I could now sleep it off. Before it had been far too painful to even contemplate sleep.

The pattern had changed. Given that this coincided with changes in hormonal patterns then I can only conclude that I, as a female, had a greater risk because of the hormones associated with being female.

This would tie in with all research which shows that being female is a risk factor for migraine. In fact, I know plenty of women who do have migraines but I know of only one male and that was my youngest son.

If I had known how debilitating migraines were I would seriously have considered not having children rather than pass the condition onto them.

I now have a great quality of life. By trial and error, I worked out the triggers for my own migraines – far more than the one or two that many medics believe are responsible. I have learned the value of ice bags and gel packs – both invaluable to me. If I was out and the beginnings of a migraine started, I would head for the nearest ice drinks and hold one to the nape of my neck. That helped delay and attenuate the condition.

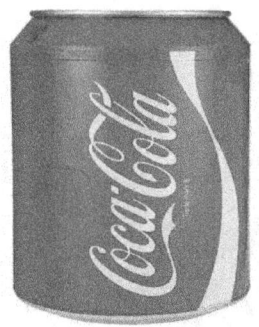

A refrigerated can of coke, rolled on the nape of the neck is wonderfully soothing

The three nutrients that made the difference to me were tryptophan, vitamin C and magnesium. I have to take these in far greater quantities than the Recommended Daily Allowance but it works and it is such a small price to pay to feel human.

Of course there are still risk factors but they do not appear to be huge risk factors anymore; it is more an understanding that I go gently with some of the foods that used to bring on migraine swiftly and some adaptations to some of the foods I enjoyed.

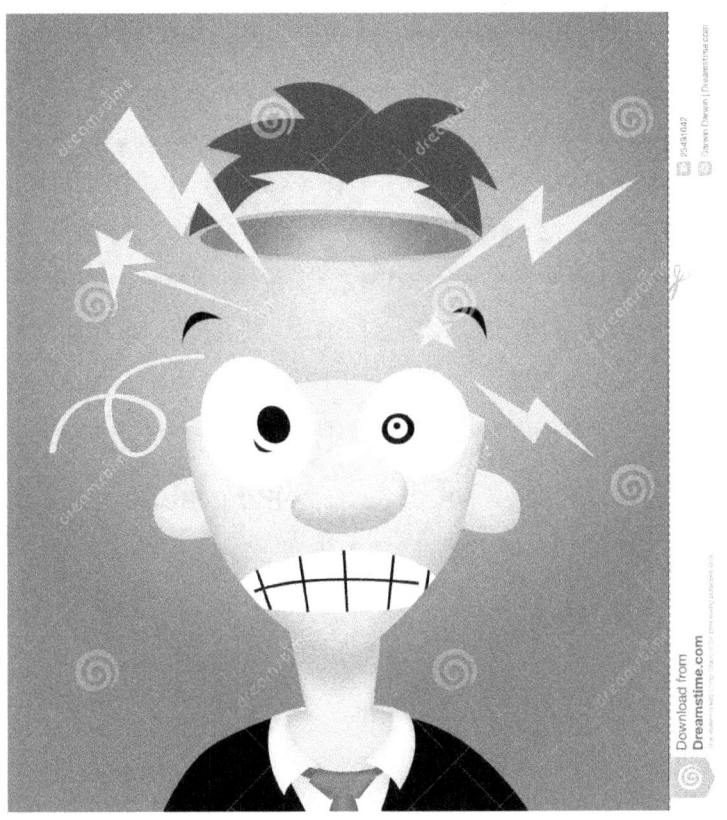

MSG can make migraineurs feel weird

Of course, everyone's journey with migraine will be personal to them. The risk factors will be different and some individuals may only have one trigger and others may have a number.

Even if there is only one risk factor – for example, hydrolysed protein, this substance is ubiquitous and avoiding it is a major task. Not everyone has the time, the skills or the patience to make a range of home- made food to store in the freezer. Now and again a little spontaneity in having a meal is welcome. I love eating out and chatting over things in a relaxed atmosphere now and again.

I don't always want to be rifling about in the freezer and eating at home.

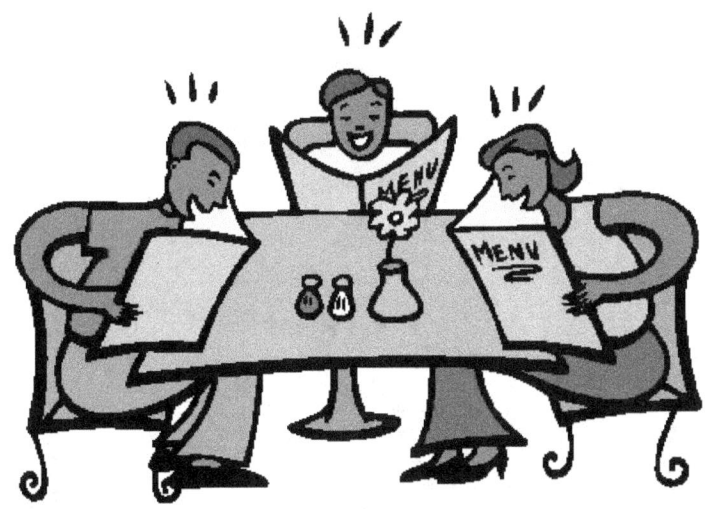

[7]Eating out and being with the mainstream can present particular challenges for those with migraine.

Like any other chronic disease such as diabetes, self-management of migraine is crucial. Being disciplined is also crucial. Veer away from avoiding the known triggers and migraine will descend quickly and mercilessly.

A bespoke action plan is a necessity. Firstly, you need to identify the triggers. This may involve keeping a food diary and looking at the foods and beverages taken in the preceding 48 hours before a migraine takes hold. However, many

---

[7] https://www.clipart.email/clipart/dining-out-clipart-21878.html

migraineurs have subconsciously sussed out what brings on a headache. The next task then is to identify what these triggers have in common. Are they high in histamines or nitrates, for example?

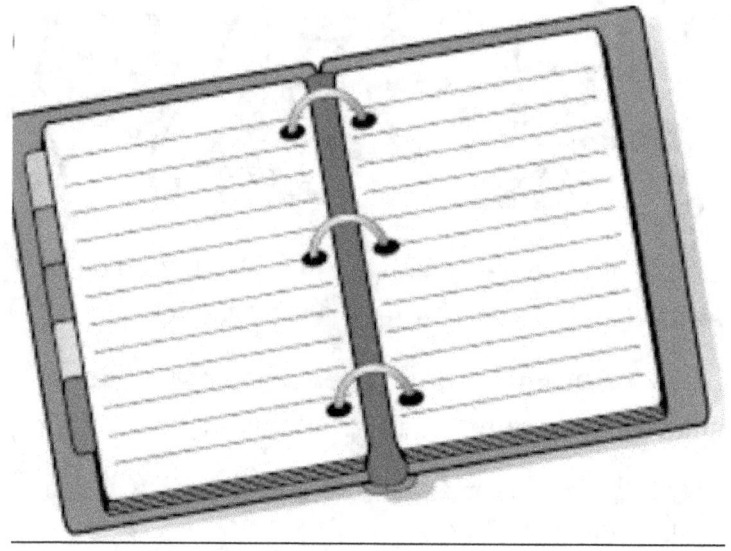

A food diary is an essential weapon in identifying food triggers for migraine.

Once the triggers have been established then avoiding them is the best bet. It may be that a small amount of the trigger food may not result in a headache while larger amounts may. This will also be subject to trial and error.

If you suffer from asthma, angioedema or urticarial (as I did until I took larger doses of vitamin C) then one of your likely triggers is histamine and a low histamine diet should be followed or an increase in the enzyme DAO which is found in olive oil may well help.

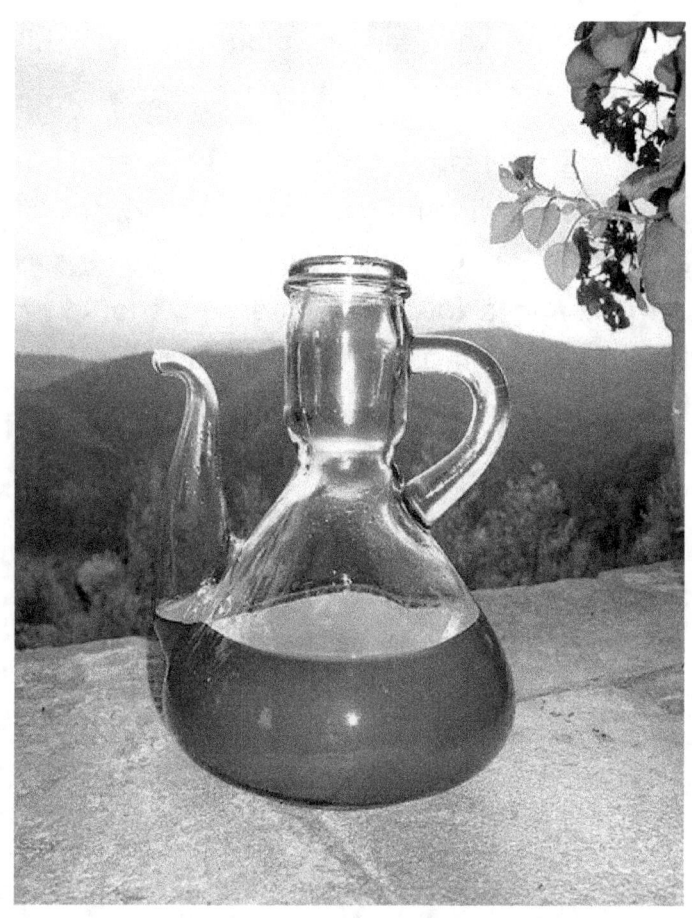

Olive oil helps reduce the effects of histamine

While antihistamines are useful in migraine one of the side effects of antihistamines is that they promote weight gain and this is unacceptable to many especially when vitamin C works just as well and aids weight loss.

A bespoke rescue pack needs to be assembled. This you must carry around with you so that you can use the contents as soon as you feel a migraine coming on.

Make sure that you have complex carbohydrates to hand. A couple of digestive biscuits carried in your bag – in much the way that diabetics, carry dextrose tablets – is prudent.

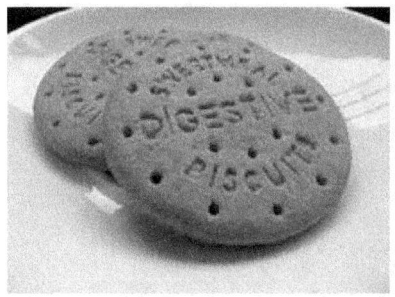

Get into the habit of carrying a couple of digestive biscuits to eat as soon as you feel a couple of migraines coming on

Buy an ice bag or crush up ice cubes and place them in a plastic bag ready to apply to the nape of your neck. Buy a gel mat which takes away the heat from dilated blood vessels.

After a while this will become a way of life that you continue almost without thinking about it.

Since this book was written, two more highly effective substances have been added, which work in different ways but, nevertheless, are excellent additions to the migraineurs medicine bag.

I have added these as extra chapters, below

Curcumin

Curcumin has become big news in the last few years as a powerful anti-inflammatory which has lasting benefits for inflammatory processes going on in the brain. It has been shown to lower the risk of Alzheimer's and has had some success in reversing some of the cognitive dysfunction that is associated with Alzheimer's disease.

Before I go any further, I should explain the difference between curcumin and turmeric as some people think it is one and the same thing.

Curcumin is the active ingredient in turmeric but there is precious little in it – certainly not enough to make a difference to an impending migraine attack.

Curcumin has to be bought separately – it often comes at a price –and for good absorption it often comes with black pepper or piperine. Curcumin is also helped if it is taken with a little fat, too.

Curcumin helps because of its superior anti-inflammatory properties which can curtail neurogenic inflammation.

A study was carried out on 44 women with migraine. The women were allocated either 500mg of curcumin twice daily or placebos. This study was 8 weeks in length.

Markers such as the concentration of the inflammatory interleukin -6 and clinical symptoms such as:

Headache severity

Duration

frequency

were measured before and at the end of the study.

At the end of the study, there was a significant reduction in the severity and duration although the frequency did not change much

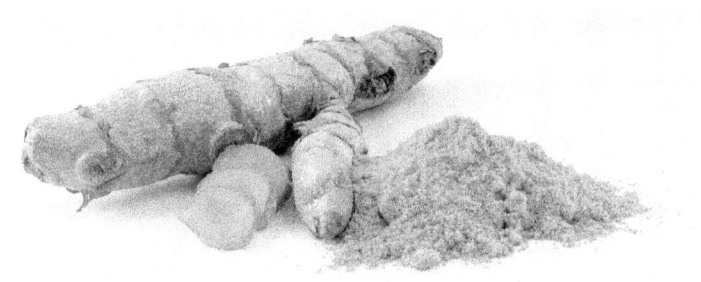

Curcumin has benefits for migraine sufferers.

We now need to look at one further vitamin in the group known as the B complex. This is vitamin B1 also known as thiamine.

In the 1930's and 1940's, thiamine was used for pain relief for those women who were in labour. It not only took the edge off the pain but it also shortened labour.

As time has gone on we have forgotten about thiamine, a miracle drug in its own right. It deserves a little more attention.

Thiamine – the righter of all wrongs

Thiamine is a minor miracle in its own right. For example, thiamine has not been found to have any upper tolerable limit, nor does it interact negatively with any other medication.

Thiamine is required for every cell in the body where it acts in the mitochondria (the power house of the cell) to provide the spark that is required for oxygen and glucose to provide energy.

The proper functioning of the mitochondria is essential in order to prevent migraine.

In order for thiamine to be activated, it requires magnesium – where would we be without this trace mineral which is so often deficient in the majority of the population?

Now, the recommended daily intake for thiamine is said to be 1.2mg. Most people become deficient very quickly on this amount as thiamine is degraded or inhibited by the use of:

Alcohol

High carbohydrate diets

Tea and coffee

And some medications like Metformin.

When thiamine deficiency occurs a condition known as beri beri occurs and this impacts three main areas of the human body:

Wet beri beri impacts the cardiovascular system

Dry beri beri impacts the nervous system

And there is a form known as gastrointestinal beriberi

These are severe conditions with long lasting impact. It can progress to Wernicke's encephalopathy and Korsakov's syndrome – generally in those who drink alcohol.

If the conditions have not been evident for a long time, reversal with vitamin B supplementation is possible although the full effect may not be seen for 3-6 months.

Other research has found thiamine's ability to address headaches in high doses. It has been found that supplementing with thiamine in doses of between 1000mg-4000mg alleviated headache in up to 78% of patients.

Another study examined 13,439 subjects who had experienced severe headache and had lower intakes of thiamine.

The results showed that there was an association between thiamine and headaches. There was a negative correlation between thiamine intake and the frequency or severity of the headache.

Women represented double the number of migraineurs than men.

Thiamine increase GABA in the brain. GABA functions by reducing neuronal excitability, thus inhibiting nerve transmission. Thus GABA reduces pain signals, reduces anxiety and insomnia by calming things down.

Always remember though that in order to take advantage of thiamine's miraculous properties you need to activate it by having enough magnesium in your diet. The more thiamine you take the more magnesium you will need.

Up to 500mg of magnesium may be needed with very high doses of thiamine. Increasing potassium (found in fruit and vegetables) as well as including a B complex all helps thiamine to function optimally.

Since I wrote this chapter's Final Thoughts, my research has taken me further and most of this chapter would be superfluous for me, now. However, I kept it in because the process and causes of migraine may vary in different individuals. As such, the information it contains may have value for some.

However, my migraine days have finally ended with the addition of extra tryptophan to my diet. I simply do not have migraines anymore.

I conclude, given the familial history, that there is a susceptibility in our genetic make-up in the serotonergic pathway. This discovery has been a long time coming but it may benefit my future generations just as it may help some readers here.

That is my hope anyway, that readers will find benefit in this book and finally be free from this debilitating condition.

Appendix

Major risk factors for migraine

- Emotional or physical stress
- Strong sensory input such as noise, strong scents or bright sunlight
- Hormonal changes
- Inconsistent eating patterns
- Inconsistent sleeping patterns
- Food and drink containing monosodium glutamate (often used in Chinese cuisine).
- Departing from a usual routine
- Low serotonin levels

Table of foods high in histamine[8]

---

[8] https://tart.tscoreks.org/histamine-chart/

LOW	MODERATE	HIGH	VERY HIGH
FRUIT Golden delicious apples, banana, pears peeled, paw paw	**FRUIT** Red delicious apples, grapefruit, kiwifruit, lemon, mango, passion fruit, pear with skin, persimmon, rhubarb, tamarillo, watermelon	**FRUIT** Apples (Granny Smith, Gala), cherries, lychee, mandarin, peach, tangelo	**FRUIT** Apricots, berry fruits, grapes, orange, plum, pineapple, rock melon, All dried fruit – dates, prunes, sultanas, raisins, etc. All jams, jellies, marmalade, fruit juices
VEGETABLES Bamboo shoots, bean sprouts, brussel sprouts, cabbage (green & red), celery, chickpeas, chives, choko, kidney beans, leeks, lentils, lettuce, lima beans, peas (fresh & dried), potato peeled, shallot, swede	**VEGETABLES** Asparagus, beans green, beetroot, carrot, cauliflower, kumera, marrow, mushroom, onion, parsnip, potato unpeeled, pumpkin, sweetcorn, turnip	**VEGETABLES** Alfalfa sprouts, broad beans, broccoli, cucumber, egg plant, spinach, watercress	**VEGETABLES** Capsicum, courgette, gherkin, olive, radish, tomato, all tomato based foods – tomato sauce, baked beans etc.
OTHER FOODS Garlic, parsley, soy sauce, malt vinegar, cashew nuts, poppy seeds, cocoa, carob, sugar, golden syrup, chocolate, camomile tea, dandelion coffee, tonic water, gin, vodka, whisk	**OTHER FOODS** Nuts, coconut, sesame seeds, sunflower seeds, beer, cider, sherry, brandy	**OTHER FOODS** Honey, marmite, vegemite, coffee, wine, port, fruit teas	**OTHER FOODS** Herbs & spices, white vinegar, Worcester sauce, tea, peppermint tea, rum, liqueurs

Thank you for purchasing this book. Every time a book is purchased, a donation is made to one of the charities I am currently supporting. One of the charities that has been supported through the sale of this book is The Exodus Project.

The Exodus Project

My first introduction to the far reaching impact of The Exodus Project occurred when I was travelling around Cawthorne in one of their buses, visiting gardens. A young lad was happily munching on a sandwich. He looked up briefly, pointed to the driver and said,' He's my second dad, he is,' then he returned to his sandwich without further comment

Such remarks are often very telling and so I arranged to meet Jackie Peel and Martin Sawdon, at the charity's premises in Barnsley. They set up the Exodus Project 20 years ago. They moved into their current premises – a redundant Methodist church - in 2010.

Both Jackie and Martin have been youth workers in their church. Martin worked in housing for the homeless in addition to working in learning disabilities services in institutional settings.

The work that the Exodus Project undertakes is of paramount importance to the communities it serves. These were former mining communities which became disadvantaged after pit-closures. Currently about 400 children attend mid-week activities from Monday to Thursday inclusive. These activities include dance, drama, craft, music, sports and games. In addition, there are weekend camps, cycle treks, outward bound activities, bowling and swimming. The children are taught valuable life skills including how to cook and bake. It is all about teaching children how to fulfil their potential and learn skills they will be able to pass onto the next generation.

The grounds, once overgrown, have been turned into a play- and camping - ground. A miniature railway is in the process of being installed.

Martin and Jackie have developed a unique model in that The Exodus Project goes beyond dispensing services. They are keen to build up relationships with the whole family and not just the child that attends the mid- week clubs. In addition, once children have reached the age of fourteen, they are invited to help out with the younger groups as junior volunteers. Once they reach the age of eighteen, they become adult volunteers. This model provides a constant supply of help from individuals who have benefitted already from attending such groups.

The building is large and inviting. It is decorated with bold colours and has comfy seating. It is a real home from home; a haven for families who have been disadvantaged by the closure of the life force of its community.

Martin and Jackie have clear ideas about how they wish to develop the Exodus Project but the lottery funding which they benefitted from is no longer available. Sadly, they have had to close two of their clubs due to lack of funding. This decision wasn't taken lightly. They do have two charity shops which raises some money and they obtain some funding from outside organisations for the use of their facilities.

However, this is clearly not enough to keep their clubs, weekend activities and building going to cater for the ever growing number of children who are benefitting from the work being undertaken here. Neither does it allow for future development.

Exodus do have a Just Giving page which can be found here if you wish to help further their work https://www.justgiving.com/exodus

In addition, you can keep up with activities on their Facebook page here

https://www.facebook.com/search/top/?q=the%20exodus%20project%20barnsley&epa=SEARCH_BOX

If anyone wishes undertake an event like The Three Peaks - or run a marathon to raise funds for Exodus - then Martin or Jackie would be pleased to hear from you. This will enable their vital work in the community to continue.

Contact them through their website to be found on www.exodusproject.org.uk.

Other Health Related Books by the Author

- The Reluctant Bowel
- A Weighty Issue
- Sleep, Perchance to Dream
- The Journey: EDS and chronic pain
- The MND diet: using nutrition to slow down the progress of neurodegeneration
- A Necessary Sorrow
- Taking another Road: Pain: its causes and what can be done about it.
- Osteoarthritis
- Treat infection naturally
- Treatment strategy for Migraine

You may also be interested in the semi-autobiographical trilogy of the authors life found in these three books

- The Prejudged
- Where the Blackbird Never Sings

- A Summer's Symphony

And the author's children's books
- Fanny and Victorian Jack
- Fanny and the Gamekeeper's Cottage

https://www.amazon.co.uk/~/e/B07BPQZ5CD

www.ingramcontent.com/pod-product-compliance
Lightning Source LLC
Chambersburg PA
CBHW051315220526
45468CB00004B/1359